DIET: A PRESCRIBED WAY OF LIFE

REFLECTIONS ON THE ART OF NUTRITION

BARBARA RUBIN

BALBOA
PRESS

A DIVISION OF HAY HOUSE

Balboa Press books may be ordered through booksellers or by contacting:

Balboa Press
A Division of Hay House
1663 Liberty Drive
Bloomington, IN 47403
www.balboapress.com
1 (877) 407-4847

Because of the dynamic nature of the Internet, any web addresses or links contained in this book may have changed since publication and may no longer be valid. The views expressed in this work are solely those of the author and do not necessarily reflect the views of the publisher, and the publisher hereby disclaims any responsibility for them.

The author of this book does not dispense medical advice or prescribe the use of any technique as a form of treatment for physical, emotional, or medical problems without the advice of a physician, either directly or indirectly. The intent of the author is only to offer information of a general nature to help you in your quest for emotional and spiritual well-being. In the event you use any of the information in this book for yourself, which is your constitutional right, the author and the publisher assume no responsibility for your actions.

Any people depicted in stock imagery provided by Getty Images are models, and such images are being used for illustrative purposes only. Certain stock imagery © Getty Images.

Print information available on the last page.

ISBN: 978-1-9822-2311-3 (sc)
ISBN: 978-1-9822-2312-0 (hc)
ISBN: 978-1-9822-2313-7 (e)

Library of Congress Control Number: 2019902473

Balboa Press rev. date: 03/11/2019

Author photo taken by Ron Tetteroo.

Translated by Translation Street

To my daughter Paulina, whose birth
made me the woman I am today.

If ever there is tomorrow when we're not together …
there is something you must always remember. You are
braver than you believe, stronger than you seem, and
smarter than you think, but the most important thing
is, even if we're apart … I'll always be with you.
—Winnie the Pooh

CONTENTS

LEGAL NOTICE

ACKNOWLEDGMENTS

The concept of this book developed over a long period and would not have come about without the help of many people who assisted, advised, and supported me. Anyone who has taken it upon him- or herself to write such a publication surely knows how difficult it is to decide which information to include.

Material gathered over time is arranged according to different criteria into various piles, which have a strange habit of constantly changing and mysteriously multiplying. Decisions already made break down under the weight of new ideas, and even the best-laid plans are thwarted.

It's not enough to merely repeat St. Thomas Aquinas's well-known prayer, "Lord, keep my mind free from the recitation of endless details; give me wings to get to the point ... Teach me the glorious lesson that occasionally I may be mistaken."

Everything seems important; it would be a shame to get rid of this or that, but something else is worth keeping. The work lasts months, even years, and your initial optimism and enthusiasm are replaced by fatigue and doubt.

Anyone who's been through this fight knows it can't be won alone. I would like to thank all the people who trusted me, guided me, and shared all my difficulties, joys, and dilemmas related to the creation of this publication. My heartfelt gratitude goes to those who made it possible for me to reach the final destination of this intellectual escapade.

I'd like to especially thank Paulina Darowska, my beloved daughter, for her unconditional love, her ability to care for someone close to her each day, for her understanding and tolerance of human frailties and moods, and for her belief in me. Thanks to you, I know that it's worth it to keep trying despite the opposition of fate.

To Alicja Bezmionow, my friend and soul sister, thank you for your long, valued, inspiring conversations; for motivating me to seek out wise solutions both in small matters and big ones; and for your brave idealism and uplifting advice, which have proved to be priceless values in my life.

To Iwona Karpińska, my loyal friend, I can be myself around you, reveal my weaknesses to you, and still have faith in your true friendship. You will always be with me.

To Corry van Wilderen, my friend, thank you for being with me in the most difficult moments of my life and for your ability to keep me in good spirits like no one else can.

I am grateful to Ruud Hiensch, my friend, who believed in me and for his broad, strong shoulders supporting me in moments of hopelessness and doubt. Thank you for your friendship and trust.

Thank you also to Anton, who served as the central driving force behind this work with admirable wisdom and patience, not only in moments of doubt, but also when it was necessary to take a calculated and essential risk or to intervene in my working methods.

While I'm at it, I'd like to extend a respectful thanks to the farmers, producers, and breeders who, fearless in the face of numerous problems and difficulties, have decided to raise organic, ecofriendly crops and oversee humanely run livestock operations. Without their efforts, any dreams of health and responsibility for the human condition would be impossible. I tip my hat to them and cry out with applause: thank goodness for them!

INTRODUCTION

My Journey

We all have those turning points in life. Call them trials, crossroads, "aha" moments, or even opportunities. These pivotal experiences tend to bring us to our knees and force us to make a choice. You either keep trudging along—even though you know in your heart something is not right—or you change.

When I was in my early thirties, I went through a life-changing health crisis. In the buildup, before my physical breakdown happened, I was, for all appearances, a healthy, successful, thriving adult. I had a busy career as a personal trainer. I was always fully booked and boasted a schedule filled with celebrity clients. I looked great. Back then, I followed the mantra of intense exercise and a low-calorie, low-fat diet—the idea that never feeling full and nourished, never letting yourself rest and indulge was the key to optimal health.

But there was a problem. A big one.

Despite all my hard work, my supposedly healthy and fit lifestyle, my quest for the *idea* of wellness and success was slowly destroying my body, mind, and spirit. And I didn't even realize it.

Right before my critical turning point, I knew something was off. I was always tired. The sun was shining, and I'd be the one fighting off a cold. I followed a strict fitness regimen, yet instead of feeling energized and alive, I felt exhausted and depressed. The pressure to embody physical perfection in my career led me to extreme dieting and neglecting what my body needed, turning food into a source of illness, not wellness. Headaches, stomach pains, PMS, sleep problems, skin issues—you name it, I was living it.

I went to plenty of doctors, trying to find out what might be wrong. They all told me I was fine. I wasn't.

When I was thirty-two, I came down with the flu but instead of getting better after a couple of weeks, I was still sick months later. Then, without warning, I experienced the worst fever of my life. My temperature went above 40° (104°F). I thought I was having a seizure it was so intense.

My skin turned white, my teeth started to chatter uncontrollably, and my body began to shake violently. I screamed out in pain, like a wolf in agony. It wasn't pretty. Even my dog hid under the bed. For the next few days, I went through a series of these high-fever episodes before it finally stopped.

From that experience, I swore to myself I was never going to be sick again. I knew my previous concept of health was all wrong; I just didn't know how or why yet. I had to start from scratch, get to the bottom of well-being, and learn how to be healthy, for real. This low was the beginning of my journey to discovering the true power of food.

I haven't been sick since.

How did I get here?

I stopped just accepting information and started digging it up myself. It began with books. I'd read anything I could get my hands on about diet, nutrition, and the evolution of food production. Then I started taking courses, traveling the world to attend health-related seminars, and talking to medical professionals—from conventional medical doctors to alternative therapists and healers—to learn what they knew.

Hormonal imbalances, digestive health, detoxification—I studied every facet of the impact of food on wellness. I discovered the works of legends such as Weston A. Price, Francis Marion Pottenger, and Roger Williams. I investigated the teachings of Charles Poliquin and wanted to start taking his courses. Then, by good fortune, fate, chance, whatever you want to call it, I stumbled upon Paul Chek and started training to become a holistic health coach. I later began working with clients.

Instead of teaching them to push their bodies as I had as a physical trainer, I was privileged to become a part of their journey, guiding them to a deeper well-being through healthy eating and a healthy lifestyle. I loved it! And I still enjoy this work immensely today.

What I discovered is, on my previous quest for perfection, I had been doing everything that I believed to be so right, so wrong—too much exercise, too many supplements, and I was totally off on my approach to food.

What I also was shocked at is how the information that *is* readily available is too thin, even misleading, making it almost impossible for busy, active individuals who want to improve their health to do so. It took a lot of effort for me to uncover what healthy eating truly means and how critical diet is not only to building a well-tuned physical body but for mental and emotional health as well.

I believe there is a standard level of modern health. We may eat our veggies and go to the gym, but we're still stressed. We still have headaches and digestive problems and feel sluggish most of the time; we simply have come to accept these symptoms as "normal." This standard level is where we are all running around, doing our best with our career, family, and health, but honestly have no idea how much each small choice in what we eat and where we source our food dictates our entire experience of life.

And then, there's this ideal level of health, where a lot of us have the desire to be and could be, quite easily, if we only knew a little more about how food impacts our physical, mental, and emotional selves.

That's why writing this book has been so important to me. I want to create that bridge from where you are today to where you can be. My intent is to provide you with the knowledge that will allow you to eat well and love it, without having to research all the science; to travel the world talking to different farmers, doctors, and food producers who have dedicated their lives to health; or to study the evolution of human beings' approach to food over the decades—unless, of course, you want to!

I want to give you the tools to begin eating an organic, clean, whole-food diet, starting today. I want to leave you inspired by the independent food producers who are preserving a sustainable way of life for all of us and awestruck at the perfect rhythm and harmony we can create in our own bodies—and our own lives—simply by becoming more aware of what we eat.

I'm forty-seven years old, and I'm healthier than ever—not just fit but full of energy and joy. I look pretty much the same as I did over a decade ago. I feel amazing and content. What I've uncovered about food isn't just for physical health. It's the key to being able to live fully and embrace life holistically.

I want to feel this way when I'm one hundred, and I know now the secret to doing this is food. My road to wellness started with changing my diet. That's what gives you the power to change everything else.

This knowledge saved my life. And that is exactly why I want to share it with you.

All the best,
Barbara

A GUIDE TO THIS BOOK

This isn't your typical book about healthy eating. Yes, it will help you improve your diet. It will inspire you and teach you how to live a healthier lifestyle through smarter food choices. But this book is more than that. It's about our *idea* of food and what role it should play in our life. It's a holistic view of nutrition itself—how the way we conceptualize food writes the story of our health and of our life.

When you are finished reading *Diet: A Prescribed Way of Life*, you'll walk away with a totally transformed perspective on food and nutrition. And you'll have the knowledge you need to make truly well-informed choices about your diet.

This isn't about counting calories. I'm not going to tell you to fill your cabinet with supplements or to try out diets that will force you to give up the foods that you love. This book is about recentering ourselves through a ruthlessly honest and science-based look at where we are today and recreating our relationship with food so we know what to eat, how to prepare it, and how to provide our bodies with the nutrition we need in order to thrive now and in the future.

Food isn't just medicine. It's the life source. That's why understanding every part of the process—from the soil your food is grown in, to the way it's cared for and how it is processed—matters. That's why reading this book matters.

It's also why I took a heavily scientific approach when writing it. This isn't a look at nutrition based on anecdotal evidence or personal experience. The knowledge in this book is based on science.

Diet also presents an objective look at nutrition, getting outside of our current food paradigm—chasing the latest diet trend or supplement only to find ourselves filling our plates with new versions of processed foods and missing out on the deep vitality that comes from a more traditional diet.

I want you to see the bigger picture—the evolving relationship of humankind with food—so you too can discover what I have learned: the power of a "prescribed way of life."

I've divided the book into two parts: Part 1 gives you a historical perspective on nutrition. It's an in-depth look at how we've gone from primitive peoples living a hunter-gatherer life to modern humans with all of our current cognitive abilities. In this part of the book, I discuss what role nutrition—especially animal protein—has played in this process. And then comes the scary part—the fact that today, in our advanced modern society with all our access to information and different types of food, our biological development has slowed down and is even reversing.

This is why this book is so critical right now: our current approach to nutrition is helping the human race *devolve*. Our brains are getting smaller. The human physique is contracting.

In the first half of the book, I look at what has happened and is happening right now that is contributing to the dwindling of the rich, physical inheritance left to us by our forbearers.

A lot of the conclusions I've uncovered may surprise you. But they are also meant to empower.

This first part of *Diet* is also intended as a reflection of what we are capable of in the future—not just what's in store if we maintain the current perspective on nutrition but also an honest look at the quality of the future existence we are heading toward.

Why the focus on evolution to understand diet and nutrition today?

This focus is critical to understanding how food has made us what we are today and how our nutritional choices now will color who we become in the future. The transitions in our evolution—the gradual appearance of hunting and farming alongside most ancient gathering cultures—point to the pivotal role animal meats and fats have played in our development as humans. Before we look at today's science on nutrition, we need to understand the key insights into anatomy, genetic makeup, and adaptability that the history of the human race and evolutionary processes reveal.

With the health issues we face today, we need this level of relevance and realism injected into the conversation on food. It's impossible to understand how we got to where we are and why we eat the way we do without a look back at the road that brought us to this point in time. I believe it's through this knowledge of evolution that we can work toward improving our quality of life and health now and in the future.

With this knowledge, we, as individual consumers, will be able to make more conscious choices about what we eat, demanding organic, humane, and ecofriendly, healthy food from farms and retailers and turning away from the foods that don't meet those standards because we know what continuing to consume them means.

Part 2 discusses the art of nutrition from a holistic perspective. It delves into the existing tension with the modern diet—the fact that what's good for us and unscrupulous consumerism are moving in opposite directions. And it strives to guide you to search for your own personalized nutrition regimen that will fuel a healthy lifestyle while developing a commonsense, relaxed approach to food.

The fact is there's no such thing as a healthy diet. The Holy Grail that other books, diet fads, and nutritional trends promise doesn't exist. That's because the "problem" doesn't exist with any specific food. It's found in how food interacts with your own body chemistry.

In order to eat well, you have to go on a personal journey. To start, you need to look at your genetic background and metabolic type to understand how your body interacts with different foods. This is the information that will help you establish the principles of your diet.

Then, you have to look at how your food is sourced and prepared. For example, healthy eating isn't about choosing red meat or fish but rather selecting organic, sustainable humane protein sources that work well for your body and choosing the right way to prepare them and the right foods to enjoy them with. It's about looking at how you serve your family and community in the process. After reading part 2, you'll know how to make these wise food choices for yourself.

Part 2 also explores the ways you can recognize what foods to eat to help yield the results you want for your health. Some foods trigger hormones that encourage fat loss or gain. Others increase the absorption of nutrients. And other foods directly support different body systems, like the immune system or your nervous system.

You'll learn how to eat right through understanding how foods affect your body, not by counting calories or relying on supplements to meet your nutritional needs. And, in the process, you'll get to fall in love with food all over again as you discover just how tasty a healthy, sustainable, whole-food diet can be.

You'll also find out what the current research says about eating chemically treated or genetically modified foods and what risks are involved when you don't know what you are putting into your body.

You'll learn the science behind healthy fats and the different ways that fresh and rancid or burned fats interact with our bodies, the benefits of real salt, and the differences between dairy products from A1 and A2 cows. Omega fatty acids, the amazing healing properties of broth, the reason you should never eat egg whites without yolks, and how the rich potency of ancient grains dwarfs the nutritional value of refined and hybrid grains—all of these gems of the science behind food are found in part 2.

And, of course, the purpose behind this book—you'll discover the power of food as a tool for healing and learn how to translate this power to your plate.

As the book closes, you'll find the motivating words that will, I hope, inspire you to take it upon yourself to learn more. This book is intended for those who are ready to decide for themselves what is right for them and who want to acquire the knowledge and skills that will allow them to improve the quality of their lives with wisdom.

If I have motivated you to walk your own journey of healthy eating, my book has been a success. You see, my intention is not to impart what I have learned but rather to arm you with the information—the science, the history, and the current models on nutrition—to help you take the next step.

As my good friend, an exceptionally wise Russian teacher and director of a well-known high school in Moscow, told me on her eighty-seventh birthday, "The best teacher is not the one who communicates information, but the one who inspires curiosity and the desire to learn." I sincerely hope my book does exactly that for you.

A WORD FROM THE AUTHOR

The word *diet* itself comes from Greek (*diaita*) and was understood as a "prescribed way of life" or "the right and proper way." After all, the ancients observed the relationships noted in the preceding section and saw that sickness and weakness are not only the result of detrimental environmental factors and twists of fate but primarily of lifestyle and the food we eat.

Observing nature, I realized that, in even the smallest form of life, with its exceptional, precise, and complex internal structure, there is a great wisdom beyond our understanding, a mysterious logic. Each life form is an extremely sensitive system that reacts to external signals and stimuli and is part of the universe itself. Consequently, changing our diet begins a process of transformation, which could then serve as the driving force for even greater change.

The history of humankind and its cultures clearly shows that dietary models based on traditional principles are the best guarantee of optimal physical and psychological health, a source of energy allowing us to survive and overcome difficulties, and a true wellspring of vital strength enabling us to work, fight, and produce healthy offspring.

Diets inspired by the rich culinary histories of cuisines around the globe offering a broad range of properly prepared, unprocessed, and organically raised foods are the best and healthiest option for your health and vitality. Nothing can take the place of homemade fish and meat broths and fresh vegetables and fruits, as well as an array of pickled foods, natural dairy products, mineral water, and fermented drinks. Each of these should be a permanent fixture of every diet in the world.

By returning to the "old ways" of eating, we stand for the values that are ignored today. While it's true that we want to live long and in good health, we'd also like that life to be dignified. As the old Roman saying goes, "If you want peace, prepare for war." Trying to fight a multitude of dietary systems that lie so far from the idea of proper, responsible, organic, and healthy nourishment may seem like Don Quixote tilting at windmills—but trust me, it's worth it!

Going back to a time in which raw, organic vegetables, fruits, and herbs were the basis of every person's diet is not only a fascinating journey but—most importantly—a healthy and nutritious one. Nothing compares to the true pleasure of eating ice cream made from fresh cream or scrambled eggs from the creation of happy chickens or the aroma of real bee honey, all of which have now been supplanted by substitutes full of aspartame, refined salt, chemical creamers meant to resemble milk, burnt powdered eggs, and other deceitful and disgusting inventions that can all be called one thing: harmful, cheap fakes.

The challenge for each of us is to determine an individual, healthy, optimal diet that will meet all of our needs and expectations but will not ruin our lives or become an onerous burden. It also shouldn't transform us into neurotic diet freaks or breathless fanatics driving ourselves, our family, and our friends to madness. Food should never be associated with worry, oppressive obligation, or anxiously weighing yourself on the scale.

It should be a source of pleasure and joy—the conscious, wise provision of what we need and deserve. No diet should devolve into obsessively counting calories or pounds or become a permanent source of stress. Our ideal, individual diet will come slowly, through keen observation of ourselves, our lifestyle, and our physical activity.

To be healthy, strong, and resilient and to enjoy a wonderfully sculpted, athletic figure, we should eat food that is not only tasty, nutritious, and digestible but also consumed in the right atmosphere and specific conditions. These include a calm environment, good company, high spirits, a well-set table, beautiful dishes, decorations, flowers, music, good conversation, and so on.

Even the best dishes prepared from traditional recipes will not lead to good health or well-being if they're consumed alone or in an atmosphere heavy with arguments, envy, resentment, vindictiveness, or bitterness. As the famous Canadian chef James Barber said, "Cooking, like sex and dancing, is a pleasure best shared." Now, the real possibilities for improving your health, condition, and well-being lie in your hands.

PART 1

OUR PRIMATE HERITAGE

Is evolution a theory, a system, or an hypothesis? It is much more: it is a general condition to which all theories, all hypotheses, all systems must bow and which they must satisfy henceforward if they are to be thinkable and true.
—Pierre Teilhard de Chardin

CHAPTER 1

WHERE DO WE COME FROM?

We have a pretty good idea of the role eating meat has played in human evolution. In 1999, researchers at the University of California, Berkeley, revealed that early humans were eating animal meat 2.5 million years ago,[1] confirming a lot of the research conducted over the past century about the relationship between human evolution and animal protein.

A meat-based diet was the norm rather than the exception when you look back to the dawn of man. It was nutrient-dense animal protein that helped early humans find enough nutrition and energy to evolve from being instinctual and living in the moment to being sociable, intelligent beings, capable of recognizing patterns, planning outcomes, and better controlling their environment.

In fact, the theory is, without an animal-protein-rich diet, we probably wouldn't have evolved into what we are today. A plant-based diet simply didn't have the complexity and density of nutrition that our bodies needed during that

---

[1]   Patricia McBroom, "Meat-Eating Was Essential for Human Evolution, Says UC Berkeley Anthropologist Specializing in Diet," *Public Affairs*, accessed July 2, 2018, https://www.berkeley.edu/news/media/releases/99legacy/6-14-1999a.html.

critical transformation period to develop our brains and to help the human body itself evolve.

In the last two centuries, scholars across the board—in evolutionary biology, paleontology, and epigenetics—have taken great pains to perfect their research methods. Thanks to their work, today, we know a lot of the details of how the natural environment, dietary habits, and behavioral factors led to the development of our species. It is through this knowledge that we can gain a profound appreciation for the power of food and our relationship to our environment to help each of us make wise choices about our individual approach to food.

Scientists from the fields mentioned have studied and continue to study life and the cultures of past generations, from the moment human beings first appeared on earth and began to produce simple tools to the present day.

The scope of their work covers an unusually broad range of time (millions of years) and space (the entire planet, both on land and in the watery depths) and is, at times, general (former societies and human groups) and anonymous (without the identity and concrete nature of names and languages).

As a result of this approach to the origins and development of our species, an enormous amount of in-depth knowledge has been gained on the subject, along with a detailed picture of the conditions under which we came into being as people: *Homo sapiens.*

For us, the most interesting age is the Quaternary Period, as the history of the birth and development of humankind is tied to this period. This is the period of *anthropogenesis,* or the formation of our species. Humans did not come into existence on earth as fully formed, perfected beings with all the psychological and physical characteristics we know today.

It was over the course of seven million[2] years of evolution that humans laboriously and persistently made their way from imperfect forms that threatened their survival toward more perfect ones guaranteeing us safety, health, and further development.

The research irrefutably demonstrates humankind's evolution from animals and our genetic ties to primates, which first appeared on earth seventy million years ago.[3] To this day, scientists disagree over the classification, taxonomy, and chronology of the genesis and evolution of humankind.

However, they do agree that ten to fourteen million and six to seven million years ago, the beings known as hominids—all anthropoid apes and our precursors (large, tailless primates)—branched out into several species.[4]

There is thus a close genetic relationship between large apes and humans (98 percent of our DNA is shared with large apes).[5] The first beings to clearly differentiate themselves by their characteristic upright posture are members of the genus *Australopithecus*.

Australopithecines first appeared in East and South Africa in the Rift Valley lake region. An expedition by French and American paleoanthropologists discovered fifty-two bones

---

[2] Mark Sisson, *The Primal Blueprint* (Malibu, CA: Primal Nutrition, 2009), 15.

[3] Jaques Marseille and Nadeije Laneyrie-Dagen, eds. *Dzieje ludzkości. Największe wydarzenia w historii świata* [The History of Humankind: The Greatest Events in World History] (Presov: Larousse, 2000), 13.

[4] Marseille and Laneyrie-Dagen, *Dzieje ludzkości* [The History of Humankind], 12–13.

[5] Marseille and Laneyrie-Dagen, *Dzieje ludzkości* [The History of Humankind], 12.

of a young female skeleton there. Finding them at the height of Beatlemania, they gave her remains the name Lucy (*Australopithecus afarensis*)—the heroine of one of the rock group's songs. Her anatomy indicates that she is closer to chimpanzees than to contemporary humans.

This prehistoric beauty is a bipedal being who walked nearly upright on two legs and had strong neck muscles, long arms, and short, massive legs. Lucy is about twenty years old, weighing 30 kilograms (66 pounds) and standing 120 centimeters tall (slightly under 4 feet). Her small head sits practically on her shoulders, and her brain takes up 400 to 550 cubic centimeters (about 24.4 the 33.6 cubic inches) of the capacity of her skull, which is only about 20 percent of that of *Homo sapiens*.[6] Lucy had mainly a plant-based diet, including leaves, fruit, seeds, roots, nuts, insects, and some small vertebrates, like lizards.

Our genus *Homo* split off from *Australopithecus* something like two million years ago,[7] and a group of three *Homo* species (*ergaster, rudolfensis,* and *habilis*), along with another hominid (*Paranthropus aethiopicus*) appeared. *Paranthropus* was a vegetarian, our immediate ancestor *H. ergaster,* known as *H. erectus,* clearly ate meat.

Homo erectus stands up straighter and has a larger cerebral cortex. Its head is supported by its spine, and neck muscles that it no longer needs to support its cranium disappear. Its upper limbs become freer due to its vertical position, and it

---

[6] Stanisław Kumat, *Niech się staną bogowie* [Let There Be Gods] (Warsaw: Nasza Księgarnia, 1963), 15.

[7] Heizer Wharton, *Ten Thousand Years from Eden,* 18.

skillfully uses them to make tools. Encephalization allows the size of its brain to reach 1,000 cubic centimeters (about 61 cubic inches) of the capacity of its skull,[8] and *H. erectus* was able to use this development to create a higher level of cultural progress.

H. erectus used universal flint tools—hand axes—to dig up edible roots from the soil, clean pelts, crush bones, process wood, and create other tools shaped like elongated spindles or slender ovals. This same *H. erectus* from 1.5 million years ago was not only able to use natural fire (volcanic lava, forest fires) but also to kindle it independently using two self-invented means: percussion and friction.[9]

This primitive human form lived in groups, which sat together by the fire and planned and delegated work and activities. They also had excellent hunting and gathering skills, which allowed them to easily transition to a new food chain. Scientists have shown that these prehistoric humans, in order to maintain an appropriate balance of energy, had to eat a varied diet.

The growth of hunter-gatherer culture greatly enriched this diet. The hunting community guaranteed a relatively systematic supply of animal protein to the body through the consumption of meat, bone marrow, animal organs, and stock from the scraps of successfully hunted animals. They ate deer, bison, some elephant and rhino, wild boar, and ibex, along with seafood and fish.[10]

---

[8]   Kumat, *Niech się staną bogowie* [Let There Be Gods], 18.

[9]   Marseille and Laneyrie-Dagen, *Dzieje ludzkości* [The History of Humankind], 20.

[10]   Heizer-Wharton, *Ten Thousand Years from Eden*, 19.

Researchers have linked this diet with the growth of the human brain, whose structure and condition was undoubtedly influenced by the omega-3 fatty acids found in animals.[11]

They also believe that this diet significantly shortened the time necessary to acquire food, thus allowing our ancestors time to contemplate their surroundings, become familiar with the natural environment, and make items such as clothes and ceramics—that is, to develop the typical foundations for human culture and civilization.

Fire played a great role in this process. The hearths of *H. erectus* were specialized: certain ones served to prepare meals, others for heating, others to frighten away predators, and the rest to light caves or shelters and, later on, to create simple tools and drive away enemies.

After a certain time, *H. erectus* began to migrate freely and camp in various regions of the world, evolving into new species and subspecies (*Homo neanderthalensis, Homo habilis, Homo sapiens*, and others). Among those mentioned, Neanderthals as an anthropological type and their culture and life are the best understood, since they left numerous and often rich traces of their existence in the form of camps in caves or buried remains. Scientists from the Senckenberg Center for Human Evolution and Palaeoenvironment (HEP) in Tübingen have studied the Neanderthals' diet. Based on the isotope composition in the collagen from the prehistoric

---

[11] C. J. Hunt, *In Search of the Perfect Human Diet* (Hunt Thompson Media, 2012), DVD.

Note: In the film *In Search of the Perfect Human Diet*, journalist C. J. Hunt examines modern diets, historical findings, the predecessors to native diets, and the evolution of the human diet in search of answers to questions regarding the epidemic of obesity and diet-related diseases.

humans' bones, they were able to show that 80 percent of the Neanderthals' diet consisted of meat (mammoths and rhinoceroses) and 20 percent vegetarian food.[12]

Scientists believe that the time when *Homo neanderthalensis*'s control of the European continent after the glaciers receded also saw the birth of modern *Homo sapiens*, who came from Africa about 100,000 to 200,000 years ago. The mass appearance of *H. sapiens* is dated to around 60,000 years BCE.[13] The latest archeological finds confirm this fact.

This incoming group was not large (2,000 to 5,000 individuals) but was able to ensure its necessary living conditions to gain the best hunting grounds and to drive the Neanderthals out. Even more impressive is the fact that only 150 members of the species left the African continent behind to start a great migration over the entire planet and reach Europe.[14]

This is the true *Homo sapiens*, now the only living species of the genus *Homo*, which, for 12,000 years, has been the undisputed king of all creatures—a rational being. A philosopher living at the turn of the sixth century and also known as St. Severin of Pavia, Boethius recognized reason as humankind's fundamental attribute. He characterized humans by the following phrase: *rationalis naturac indyvidua substantia*, an individual substance of a rational nature.

---

12 *ScienceDaily*, "Neanderthals Diet: 80% Meat, 20% Vegetables," accessed April 17, 2018, https://www.sciencedaily.com/releases/2016/03/160314091128.htm.

13 Sisson, *The Primal Blueprint*, 15.

14 The "origin of man" and "out of Africa" theories find their source in Charles Darwin's *The Descent of Man*, which was later updated by Christopher Stringer and Peter Andrews and is strongly supported by the latest mitochondrial DNA studies.

Scientists studying the individual stages of humanity's origins were interested in various aspects of the lives of our predecessors. Numerous test samples have been taken at Jonas Cave in France's Auvergne region, which contains the remains of both Neanderthals and contemporary humans. These samples allowed multifaceted specialized studies to be carried out at the molecular anthropology lab at the Max Planck Institute for Evolutionary Anthropology in Leipzig. The researchers have made several important discoveries.

It turns out that our ancestors were much taller than we were and had surprisingly healthy teeth and extremely strong bones. Their diet was dominated by animal-based foods, which is shown by the numerous discoveries of bones buried near their settlements. Archeologists have found the bones of large animals, such as bison, elk, reindeer, horse, and ibex, suggesting skilled communal hunting.[15]

Studies of the human skeleton from that distant time demonstrate that our predecessors were primarily meat-eaters, while no bone evidence has been found to suggest vegetarianism among our ancestors.

Their migrations, lifestyle, daily activities, and, above all, the quality and structure of their skeletons all point to their fantastic physical condition.

The damaging and life-threatening diseases and ailments that afflict people today were completely unknown to them. Their awareness, imagination, and ability to make connections also show that our ancestors were rational beings.

---

[15]   Heizer-Wharton, *Ten Thousand Years from Eden*, 20.

Already 45,000 years ago, they were creating musical instruments and using them for artistic purposes. They created a system of communication—language—in order to logically and clearly convey important information. They were also able to imagine life after death: they were the only beings to bury their dead, equipping them for their eternal journey with useful objects, clothes, weapons, and ornaments.

A significant number of anthropologists suggest that the human species reached the evolutionary peak of its biological development around 10,000 years ago.[16] This hypothesis is supported by the musculature, skeletal structure, and size of the cerebral cortex of our ancestors. We existed in a form and condition perfectly shaped by nature!

It's not possible to present a short overview of the complex, lengthy, and fascinating process of evolution without skipping over a fair amount of interesting information and detailed research. However, they are beyond the scope of this book and are not necessary for our purposes.

Despite the fascinating and unbelievably effective way we've survived as the solitary human species for thousands of years, thanks to the logic of evolution, we should still remember that "The border separating life from death is a narrow one. The unbelievable delicacy of our body brings to mind a vision: a sort of fog condenses into human form, lingers a moment and then dissipates" (Czesław Miłosz, *A Year of the Hunter*).

---

[16]   Hunt, *In Search of the Perfect Human Diet*, DVD.

Remember

- Our bodies were shaped by over seven million years of evolution, consistently moving toward more and more perfect forms.
- The research irrefutably demonstrates humans' evolution from animals and our genetic similarity to primates: 98.4%.
- Our ancestors overcame a variety of obstacles over their long course of development to keep our species strong and healthy—contemporary humans should respect and care for this unique identity.
- The human species has been omnivorous for millions of years—our varied diet has included animal organs, animal meat, fish, and eggs, supplemented with root vegetables, grains, leafy greens, fruits, and berries.
- Researchers have linked an animal-protein-rich diet with the growth of the human brain, whose structure and condition was undoubtedly influenced by the omega-3 fatty acids found in animals.

CHAPTER 2

THE NATURAL TREASURE OF HOMO SAPIENS ... CONTINUED?

It is not the most intellectual of the species that survives;
it is not the strongest that survives; but the species that
survives is the one that is able best to adapt and adjust
to the changing environment in which it finds itself.
—Charles Darwin[17]

Treasure—that's what I'd call these bodies of ours passed
down from our ancestors; they are a wonderful example
of the painstaking, long-term influence of natural factors.
Innumerable small genetic mutations, the development of
defense and adaptive mechanisms, natural selection, the
need to maintain the species—all of these not only kept our
forebears safe in a hostile environment but allowed them to
overcome unimaginably difficult and dangerous conditions,
resulting in their gradual occupation of the entire earth.
They survived the dangerous ice ages of the Quaternary
Period, adapted to the warming of the atmosphere in the

---

[17] Often attributed to the famous scientist, but there is no substantive evidence
that Darwin said or wrote this statement.

Neolithic Period, and were able to function independently of a changeable climate.

So why is it that, after 10,000 to 12,000 years, we've begun to lower our level of biological development, reversing the process? It has been observed that our brain is now shrinking, and our physique is abruptly contracting.[18] What's going on with this rich inheritance left to us by our forebears? Let's see if we can find some answers to these questions together by carefully analyzing this bewildering phenomenon.

Researchers say that this state of affairs has been influenced by two fundamental factors. The first was our consciousness and creative capacity, which were formed over thousands of years as a result of our brain functions. They allowed us to develop our unique civilization ever more effectively and skillfully. Thanks to the use of tools, fire, weapons, and shelters, we tamed our natural environment and gained control, though not always successfully, over the natural phenomena of our surroundings.

Traits triggered by changes in lifestyle set in. The deer's agility, the wolf's fangs, and the slender frames of wild cats ceased to impress us and be regarded as examples to aspire to. Our role models were replaced by hunting tools we invented and created ourselves—the spear, atlatl, harpoon, snares— thanks to which we could hunt the animal we desired without our former effort and with minimal movement. Finally, and most important, fire allowed us to cook fresh meat, plants, grains, and fish. It has been said that "when we learned to

---

[18]   Hunt, *In Search of the Perfect Human Diet*, DVD.

cook is when we became truly human."[19] Roasted, boiled, and smoked foods radically changed the human diet and made it possible to store some for later consumption.

According to Erich Fromm, the twentieth-century German philosopher, sociologist, psychologist, and psychoanalyst, the end of our beginning arrived when humans began to realize they were alive—when life became conscious of itself. Every animal (we, of course, belong to that kingdom) lives in accordance with the laws of nature, in harmony with it.

It's not aware that it is alive or even of what it is. It doesn't understand the significance of passing time and doesn't know that the past existed and that the future awaits. It has no idea that it will die; it exists in the here and now, without guilt or shame, without plans or the need to create.

We humans are a unique sort of being[20] that is conscious of its own existence, making us an oddity of nature. We are the only species to have become disconnected from and to violate all of nature's laws![21]

The second and perhaps most important factor in the history of the human race, which completely and irrevocably changed our lives, was a universal and bloodless economic

---

[19]   Michael Pollan, *Cooked*, Netflix Documentary Series (Netflix, 2016). Official description: "Explored through the lenses of the four natural elements—fire, water, air, and earth—*Cooked* is an enlightening and compelling look at the evolution of what food means to us through the history of food preparation and its universal ability to connect us."

[20]   This distinction is not as clear-cut as we once thought, however. As Michael Pollan notes, "One by one, science is dismantling our claims to uniqueness as a species, discovering that such things as culture, tool making, language and even possibly self-consciousness are not the exclusive domain of *Homo sapiens*" ("An Animal's Place," *New York Times Magazine*, November 10, 2002).

[21]   This view was presented by the scholar in his well-known work *The Sane Society* in 1955.

revolution: the appearance of agriculture. Around 10,000 years ago, we transformed from hunter-gatherers to beings who cultivated the land. Hunter-gatherers settled in villages on the Euphrates and Jordan Rivers 8,000 years ago, clearing the forested areas and planting grain, specifically wheat and barley. They also knew how to breed animals: sheep, goats, cows, and pigs.[22] Agriculture demands a settled way of life. Waiting for the prepared and sown fields to yield a crop requires time and patience.

Such a change in lifestyle led to a baby boom and increased competition for new farming areas when the need to leave depleted fields arose. Some of the farmers then went out to conquer new lands.

They created temporary settlements that quickly transformed into villages. These phenomena marked the beginning of the degradation and demise of the natural environment starting around 6,000 BCE. The agricultural revolution changed the world and allowed civilization, culture, technology, medicine, and many other fields of life and science to develop at an astonishing rate.

The pioneers of agriculture contributed to a change in humankind's basic diet, as the meat of raised animals and the grain harvested from the fields became a permanent part of the daily human diet. The primary mechanisms of natural selection, which had driven humankind's evolution for millions of years—the threat of hunger and danger of being caught by a predator (only the fittest should survive!)— were thus minimized. From that point on, evolution was

---

[22]   Jerzy Głosik, *Przygoda z archeologią* (Warszawa: Nasza Księgarnia, 1987), 92.

14

stopped in its tracks in a sense, and the once-strong biological tendency toward perfection ceased to have any effect.

Remember

- It was humans who spurned the timeless laws of nature and consciously ceased to live in harmony with it.
- We can stop the decline of our bodies, since we have an influence over what happens to them.
- Our mental and physical state depends on an appropriate and well-selected diet.
- Our indifference to the devastation of the natural environment will come back to bite us.
- Civilization and technology are not our enemies. When used appropriately, they can even become our allies.

CHAPTER 3

WHERE ARE WE HEADED?

In order to believe that our society has "progressed," we
must believe first that the lives of our ancestors were
indeed nasty, brutish and short. But, as study after
study has confirmed, the health of traditional peoples
was vastly superior to that of modern industrial man.
—Sally Fallon

This question reveals not only curiosity about the future of
humankind and our life here on earth but, above all, concern
over the quality of this future existence. At the turn of the
twentieth century, various predictions have been made on
this topic.

Our distant ancestors used the best, most effective, most
efficient, and most useful parts of their genetic potential to
survive. They did whatever they had to do to stay alive and be
able to propagate. Unfortunately, there are no other options.

For inexplicable reasons, contemporary humans tend to
ignore this issue. They perhaps think that, since nature gave
them this wonderful constitution for free, that it doesn't
deserve any special care.

Let's try to get a better sense of the phenomenon we are currently witnessing. I will give you some figures that stand as the clearest proof of the processes taking place.

The American National Center for Health and Statistics stated in its latest report on the state of the health of its citizens that one in three people die of cancer, one in three suffer from allergies, and one-fifth suffer from some mental illness. And that's not all! Genetic diseases, joint inflammation, multiple sclerosis, digestive disorders, diabetes, osteoporosis, Alzheimer's disease, epilepsy, chronic fatigue, and autoimmune diseases affect a significant share of the civilized population. For example, it is predicted that Alzheimer's disease will affect 106 million people by 2050. It is now the sixth leading cause of death.[23] In addition to its effects on quality of life, this terrible memory-wasting disease carries a tremendous societal cost: $60 billion a year.[24] The incidence of diabetes has increased by more than 700 percent over the last half century! At least 29 million Americans have been diagnosed with type 2 diabetes, with another 86 million considered prediabetic.[25]

As of July 2018, the world's population was estimated at 7.6 billion.[26] The United Nations currently estimates a further

---

[23] "Leading Causes of Death," Centers for Disease Control and Prevention, National Center for Health Statistics, accessed June 2, 2017, https://www.cdc.gov/nchs/fastats/leading-causes-of-death.htm.

[24] Dr. Mark Hyman, "Diabetes & Alzheimer's—The Truth about 'Type-3 Diabetes' and How You Can Avoid It" (PDF), accessed via http://drhyman.com/alzheimers/.

[25] Dr. Mercola, "The Deliberate Lies They Tell about Diabetes," Mercola.com, accessed April 20, 2016, http://www.mercola.com/diabetes.aspx.

[26] Accessed July 3, 2018, http://www.worldometers.info/world-population/?.

increase to 11.2 billion by the year 2100.[27] Each minute, 250 children are born, and 105 people die.[28] This is a baby boom without precedent in the history of humankind!

By 1000 BCE, the world was home to only 50 million people. By the first half of the nineteenth century, that number ballooned to just under one billion. Two centuries later and we have 7.6 billion people on the planet. Unfortunately, the rapidly increasing numbers have come with a heavy price. We are more susceptible to threats to our health than ever before. Public health experts believe we are at a greater risk of experiencing large-scale outbreaks and global pandemics like those we've seen in recent years: SARS, swine flu, Ebola, and Zika.[29]

On one hand, modern medicine and advancements in technology have made it possible for people to live longer lives. But, in our quest for longevity, we've overlooked the simple yet powerful things that support our health and quality of life along the way. As a result, we're living longer, but our bodies are falling apart anyway. In most developed countries today, one of society's greatest challenges is coping with growing aging populations. More and more people are developing Alzheimer's disease or other forms of dementia or illnesses that leave us unable to care for ourselves, let alone really live

[27] "World Population Prospects, the 2015 Revision," United Nations Department of Economic and Social Affairs, Population Division, accessed September 15, 2016, https://esa.un.org/unpd/wpp/DataQuery/.

[28] "World Birth and Death Rates," Ecology.com, accessed December 7, 2016, http://www.ecology.com/birth-death-rates/.

[29] Meera Senthilingam, CNN, "Seven Reasons We're at More Risk than Ever of a Global Pandemic," accessed May 17, 2018, https://edition.cnn.com/2017/04/03/health/pandemic-risk-virus-bacteria/index.html.

life. We've come to expect an almost helpless state in those last years of life as something that is normal and even anticipated and planned for.

Warnings of this health paradox began to appear from some of the greatest scientific authorities in the twentieth and twenty-first centuries. Erich Fromm, mentioned earlier in our discussion, posed the provocative question, "Must we produce *sick* people for us to have a *healthy* economy?"

Francis Fukuyama, an American philosopher, economist, futurologist, and author of numerous scientific and popular science publications, not only tells us to consider whether our health *in itself* is satisfactory but bravely reveals, "I announce the end of mankind." He is the author of the book *The Posthuman Future*, which has been recognized as an important alarm for humanity. Where did this shocking prognosis come from?

Contemporary technology, pharmacology, medicine, and biology have given humans opportunities that can't be overstated. Yet, despite the lightning pace at which the biological sciences have developed, the threats that could destroy humanity have not been eliminated.

This isn't about guaranteeing immortality, as that can't be expected from civilization, nor is it about the realization of Aldous Huxley's theory that one can create through technology a "brave new world," where, after taking the right pill, we can become happy slaves, eager to obey another person's will. In such a standardized society, nobody would even care about their own individual health.

I don't wish to give the impression that I scoff at the achievements of biotechnology, medicine, and genetics. They stand as absolute proof of the wonderful creativity and limitless possibilities of humankind and are signs of our times. I only wish to note that they are not a cure-all for the weakening of the human organism and its threatened physical condition.

In fact, on our narrow-minded mission to control our environment and our bodies, the world has gotten *more* out of control. We are facing a long list of crises—melting glaciers, polluted food sources, regular superstorms strong enough to obliterate local economies, mass exoduses of environmental and political refugees, religious and ethnic struggles that seem as if they will never end, and the turning away from those in need on a global scale.

Despite our preoccupation with sickness and health, we are sicker than ever. We may have eradicated some illnesses, only to welcome others and to subject our bodies to a life of toxic exposure and food choices that harm them. In many cases, it is our medicine that weakens us and our food that pollutes us, pushing our bodies out of their rhythms and fostering a new wave of chronic diseases like diabetes, heart disease, arthritis, chronic fatigue, and allergies.

Humans have become too bold in our desire to play God, disregarding natural laws and denying the power of the natural world to heal, support, and strengthen the individual *and* the whole. And, at the same time, we've become too complacent, immersing ourselves in the rigid structures of a postindustrial, postdigital world and forgetting our own place within the rhythm of the planet we all call home.

Are We Prolonging Our Lives or Our Agony?

Before we solve this dilemma, let's look at the results of some of the studies on the length and quality of our lives, gathered from all over the world as part of the PURE project and analyzed by, among others, Professor Salim Yusuf[30] of McMaster University in Hamilton, Canada. Ten thousand years ago, the average human life span was about thirty-three years. You may rightly notice that, compared with present-day standards, this figure is not terribly impressive!

However, it turns out that prehistoric humans lived longer than their civilized descendants up until the beginning of the twentieth century. The average life span was at its lowest during the Bronze Age (3300–1200 BCE) and Ancient Egypt: a mere eighteen years. It clearly rose again during the time of Ancient Greece (500–300 BCE) and Rome (0–500 CE), fluctuating between twenty and thirty years of age.

In the later centuries of the modern era, from the Middle Ages (500–1500 CE) to the beginning of the twentieth century, people in Europe lived to be thirty to forty years old.[31] The situation changed dramatically in the twentieth century and at the turn of the twenty-first century, because of the dynamic and never-before-seen developments in medicine, biotechnology, hospital networks, and the consciously directed health policies of many states. Yet, the average life span continues to provoke numerous controversies and is a cause for concern in many countries.

---

30   Dr. Yusuf's studies cover eighty-three countries on all the inhabited continents of the world.

31   Sisson, *The Primal Blueprint*, 17.

According to a new ranking by the World Health Organization, life expectancy in the United States rose in 2015 to 79.3 years, putting the country thirty-first in the world in terms of life expectancy. The news is a little better for women, a little worse for men. Life expectancy for females is 81.6 years; for males, this figure is 76.9 years. Australia, meanwhile, boasts a life expectancy of 82.8, putting it in fourth place worldwide. Canada comes in twelfth, with 82.2 years, with women living on average four years longer than men. The average life expectancy in Europe differs between the countries. For example, in Switzerland, life expectancy goes as high as 83.36 years, putting the country second in the world, and in Poland, it is 77.52, putting it in forty-first place. In European Union countries, women live on average seven and a half years[32] longer than men, though this is not due to genetic differences between the sexes. Geneticists and gerontologists state that if women can live longer, then it is biologically possible for men to do so as well.

Social, cultural, and mental factors all play an important role, and fortunately, those are things we can influence. This can be seen unusually clearly in the cases of the Netherlands, Finland, and Sweden. In the 1960s, the statistics were similar for Europe as a whole, but Finland had the highest mortality rate at the time. Thanks to a change in diet and the promotion of a healthy lifestyle (a campaign over a mere twenty years), deaths due to ischemic heart disease fell by 60 percent. Finnish statistics for 2013 note, "The longer life expectancy is visible in the age distribution of deaths. People are dying at

---

[32]   *The European Health Report 2012: Charting the Way to Well-Being* (Copenhagen: World Health Organization Regional Office for Europe, 2012), 6.

an ever older age: nearly two in three were aged over 75 and one in three were over 85. Four hundred of those who died had turned 100."[33]

The Finns thus planned and achieved a decline in mortality. "This is an example of how health ... can be improved or ruined," notes Professor Witold Zatoński from the Cancer Center and Institute of Oncology in Warsaw.

These results have not lessened humanity's fascination with life, the passage of time, growing old, death, and their own physical condition. Humans have noticed and continue to notice the impermanence of the world and their place in it, following the well-known principle of the French Renaissance writer and philosopher Michel de Montaigne "to know oneself, and to know how to live and die well."

How can this be done? Dr. Richard G. Cutler, a molecular gerontologist and expert on the problem of longevity, has analyzed human remains and ancient excavations and has shown that the maximum life span of our ancestors 15,000 years ago was a whopping ninety-four years! Obviously excluding any external, objective obstacles that awaited them, such as sudden accidents, injuries, and attacks by predators and enemies, he confirmed that the biological potential of the human organism guaranteed them a longer life span than that of contemporary humans by three years (91+3)[34].

The most important conclusion of his work was even more striking: they were free of the diseases that today we consider

---

[33] "Causes of Death in 2013," Statistics Finland, accessed March 1, 2017, http://www.stat.fi/til/ksyyt/2013/ksyyt_2013_2014-12-30_kat_001_en.html.

[34] Sisson, *The Primal Blueprint*, 35.

normal for our species and typical for a certain period of our lives!

What did they do better? What magical knowledge did they take to their ancient graves?

In search of the relationships between what those ancient folks ate and how they lived and died, researchers are gradually uncovering what has long been hidden in the mists of the past. A significant number of esteemed scientists, including Dr. Boyd Eaton, professor of anthropology at Emory University in Atlanta and author of *The Paleolithic Prescription*, and James V. Neel of the University of Michigan Department of Genetics, confirm that our uncivilized predecessors had the same hormonal makeup as we do, and our genetic makeup has a 99.8% overlap with that of our ancestors of 200,000 years ago.

With such recognized facts, it is easy to predict the conclusions. In spite of our awareness of the passage of time and the changes occurring around us, our basic needs (food, movement, sex, vitality, rest, and so on) haven't changed over those 200,000 years.

Humans should remember, without a hint of hypocrisy, that our origins are tied to the animal kingdom and that each creature's functioning depends on his or her primal instincts encoded within the genes, which have been passed down over generations.

Nature has equipped us with an ideal defense system to protect us from damaging external agents. Yet, alongside the development of civilization, humans are ruining the harmony created by Mother Nature and have the attitude of being above her. We've forgotten her ancient laws, carelessly rejecting them.

Like a stubborn child, humankind does everything in its power to prove to its surroundings that it can do things differently. Our eating habits, recreational activities, technical mobility, and lack of natural movement are all immense challenges not only for the immune system but also for contemporary medicine and nutritional science.

Now, it may seem as if I'm rejecting the achievements of twenty-first-century civilization. Nothing could be further from the truth! I'm not trying to convince you to give up the comfortable lifestyle that humankind has developed. What is most important is to remember and be able to use what has worked without fail for seven million years.

Despite the modern nature of our surrounding world, humans have remained basically the same. So then, why shouldn't a diet that was used over the millions of years of our species' evolution work in the twenty-first century?

After all, what was good enough in the past could also turn out to be effective today and for another seven million years as well! I like the American maxim here: "If it ain't broke, don't fix it!"

Since the riches just mentioned come from the past, I will refer to them again in the words of Michel de Montaigne:

> The great and glorious masterpiece of man is
> to live appropriately … There is nothing so fine
> and legitimate as well and duly to play the man;
> nor science so arduous as well and naturally
> to know how to live this life; and of all the

infirmities we have, it is the most savage to despise our being ... It is an absolute and, as it were, a divine perfection, for a man to know how loyally to enjoy his being ... and when seated upon the most elevated throne in the world, we are but seated upon our buttocks.[35]

Don't these words still ring true, despite being written over four hundred years ago? At each stage of our lives, we can introduce changes and cease to live just any old way. Simply going through the motions can sometimes be quite costly. Living truly healthily and well is the only worthwhile course of action!

Remember

- The Paleolithic period fed around 100,000 generations; people were slender and healthy then and practically disease-free. The agricultural era covers 600 generations, while the industrial era has lasted only ten, and people are now overweight and attacked by diseases that previously didn't exist.
- We're not hunter-gatherers anymore, so we shouldn't just blindly follow our ancestors' example. There are great lessons to be learned from what they ate and how they moved, but what keeps us alive these days is different from what allowed our caveman ancestors to

---

[35] Michel de Montaigne, "Of Experience," *Essays*, translation based on the Cotton translation by A. C. Kibel, https://ocw.mit.edu/courses/literature/21l-002-2-foundations-of-western-culture-ii-renaissance-to-modernity-spring-2003/readings/lec4.pdf.

survive: our ability to learn, process, understand, and adopt all the great knowledge of our past; our ability to master complex technological skills and absorb new information; and—most importantly—our ability to put it all together.

- Our basic needs (food, movement, sex, vitality, rest, and so on) haven't changed over 200,000 years.

CHAPTER 4

"WHAT WE HAVE BEEN OR ARE TODAY WE SHALL NOT BE TOMORROW"

It is not enough to have a good mind;
the main thing is to use it well.
—Rene Descartes

The destruction of our planet and the degradation of our natural environment seem (despite many warnings) to be accelerating at a dramatic rate. One of the justifications for this is *progress*, a word often brought up in both local and global contexts. The generator of this progress is not some mysterious, unknown power, but humans themselves, who, paradoxically, are also its victims.

When and how one could reach such depths of contempt for the laws of nature is difficult to determine today. The absurdity of the situation lies in the fact that people seem to behave as carelessly as children in such fundamental matters.

The French philosophers of the Enlightenment drew later generations' attention into the matter and dehumanized nearly all fields of study. René Descartes (1596–1650), who introduced rational dualism to that which had appeared as a harmonious whole for centuries, played a great role in this effort.

He separated the body from the soul and, with complete confidence, entrusted the former (being inert matter) to scientists and left the latter (the cast-off soul) to the realm of religion, belief, and feeling.

These days, people seem to be disoriented by this philosophical legacy and feel crippled by rationalism. It's high time we returned the soul to the body and vice versa, as one cannot exist without the other.

After all, even the best car can't run without an engine, and an engine without a car becomes a useless hunk of metal. It's time to return to a traditional, wise philosophy that sees us as beings combining physical, emotional, intellectual, and spiritual aspects into a unique, perfect whole. One can't achieve a good state of mind and health without taking this holistic principle into account.

With Hippocrates at their fore, the Greek founders of medicine considered life to consist of our psychological and spiritual development in good physical health—until our death. We have been shaped by biology and evolution to be able to live to between 120 and 130 years of age, while still maintaining our physical and psychological fitness and deriving joy from our existence.

As a holistic lifestyle coach, I have nothing but respect and admiration for the methods and principles of holistic medicine. I appreciate how such medicine stays true to the Hippocratic oath and respects the laws of nature.

Such an attitude toward Mother Nature is a source of wisdom. With full awareness and humility, I try to follow this approach and use it in both my personal life and my work with clients, encouraging them to actively take part in health-promoting activities.

We humans have been able to survive in a constantly changing environment thanks to our exceptional ability to adapt. This process took place slowly and regularly: our genetic structure has changed by a mere 0.5% over a million years.

Physically speaking, then, we are practically identical to our primitive ancestors, while we live in a completely different environment and have built a civilization straight out of a science fiction film. Despite such drastic changes, we somehow manage to survive, although this is becoming increasingly difficult.

The past hundred years are no cause for optimism, however, as we can see a huge dissonance between us and Mother Nature. I fear that the words of the Roman poet Ovid may now in fact be an ominous warning: "What we have been or are today, we shall not be tomorrow."

The changes in our surroundings reveal a contradiction and disparity between us and our environment, which has ceased to correspond to our body and our genes. The laws of nature have become completely detached from the insatiable consumerism of seven billion people who desire to possess, use, live, and, above all, eat. People currently get 70 percent of their energy from food that did not exist before. They eat and eat ... but what?

PART 2

A TABLE LADEN WITH TEMPTATION AND ILLUSION REFLECTIONS ON THE ART OF NUTRITION

There is no such thing as a healthy diet, and there has never been. There is nothing intrinsically healthy or unhealthy about any given food. All that matters is how well a particular food or dietary regimen can fulfill your unique, genetically inherited metabolic requirements.
—William Wolcott

CHAPTER 5

FOOD: AN UNKNOWN MINEFIELD

To make the right food choices, you first need to learn a bit about the subject. Most people don't differentiate between good, nutritious food and the bad stuff. They also don't realize how our body reacts to the food we eat, how it functions afterward, or what it needs to stay in good working order. Thoughtlessness and absurdity—in addition to ignorance—also play a role in our decisions regarding food.

In many other situations, we are able to exercise caution and question what we see and hear. We read the user's manuals for the televisions, computers, cell phones, and so on that we buy, and we check the warranty conditions of our newly acquired cars.

So, let's take a moment to examine our conscience, taking into account the crucial aspect of our daily lives that is the food we eat. Most of us will conclude that our poor understanding of the principles of proper nutrition is due to our lack of interest in the topic. After all, up to this point, we've only thought in terms of satisfying our hunger rather than sensible consumption and proper growth.

Many people don't realize how everything we eat influences our energy level and our physical, mental, and spiritual state.

When we stock our refrigerators and when we serve our meals, we are moving through a veritable minefield that we didn't even know was there! In our ignorance, we have no idea of the enormous difference between whole and refined grains, between hybrid and ancient grains, between traditional fresh fruits and vegetables and those which have been irradiated or chemically treated and genetically modified, between fresh fats and rancid and burnt ones, or between meat from pasture-raised animals and from those raised in suffocating, cramped cages.

Do we see that supplying food has ceased to be the simple fulfillment of the most fundamental human need and instead has turned into a ruthless, cynical business, in which financial profit has become more important than both human health and the principle of do no harm? Each time we eat and drink this or that, we unleash an avalanche of reactions and a storm of hormonal activity that influences the state of our body and mind! Unfortunately, there can be no compromises here.

"Man is what he eats," said the German philosopher Ludwig Andreas Feuerbach. I quote his opinion here to serve as our motto when we are deciding what to eat, so that we are encouraged to treat ourselves more seriously and act more responsibly when it comes to our health.

It may be easier to conceive of eating as more than a sensual pleasure if we think about the fact that millions of cells die every second and millions of new ones move in to take their place with each subsequent second. For example,

- your skin renews itself in thirty days
- your liver cells need 150 days to regenerate

- your stomach lining needs only four days to regenerate
- your intestines take two to three days to regenerate
- your fingernails renew themselves every six to ten months
- your red blood cells, which deliver oxygen to every part of your body, are replaced every 120 days
- ninety-eight percent of our body (including the skeleton!) is renewed over the course of a year[36]

All the cells in our body are like perfect microcomputers programmed to run two related, specific, and extremely important functions: maintaining optimal health and fitness at all costs and building and reconstructing what has been damaged or weakened.

We food consumers are responsible for providing the raw materials and products necessary to perform these fundamental tasks.

None of us would like to live in a high-rise built by a bunch of amateurs who just slapped it together any old way

---

[36] "In Quantum Healing, 1986, Chopra gave us a new paradigm for how the body handles its own rejuvenation processes. How often does the body renew itself? Older wisdom had it pegged at around seven years. Chopra has revised that estimate downward to roughly one year (approximately 98% totally renewed). Based on the estimates of quantum biology, you have a brand new stomach lining every 4 days, new skin every 30 days, a new liver in 6 weeks, even the skeleton is replaced every three months. These concepts are vital as we structure the metaphors for treatment while we work with our clients in the healing process."
From: "How Do Quantum Physics and Addiction Interact?" December 24, 2008, http://www.encognitive.com/node/1955. See also Benjamin Radford, "Does the Human Body Really Replace Itself Every 7 Years?" April 4, 2011, http://www.livescience.com/33179-does-human-body-replace-cells-seven-years.html.

using any old construction materials. That's obvious, right? Before you read the next section, try to remember what you've eaten over the past year, yesterday, and today.

Perhaps Ludwig Andreas Feuerbach was right: under various circumstances, our weak will can sometimes become strong, and we can introduce an exemplary diet into our lives. Exemplary, appropriate, healthy, proper—meaning what kind, exactly?

After all, as the Roman philosopher Lucretius said, "What is food to one man is bitter poison to others." So then, what should we choose?

Lost in a Maze of Diets?

The creators of many diet programs assure us that following their rules will guarantee weight loss, increased energy, a better complexion, shiny hair, and so on. We've gotten used to the loudmouthed style of these advertisements. We've become distrustful and continually sense the manipulation and lies in them that aim to separate us from our money.

How can you avoid the unreliable information of pseudoscientists and stop worrying about who's trying to convince you this time to buy these, but not those, food products? After all, nobody wants to be conned, especially since that dubious pleasure can only be had by spending one's hard-earned money.

Step 1 for any dietary changes is establishing your own personal (and very individual) metabolic type or the way your body processes food. There's no one diet or food product that's perfect and recommended for everyone.

Ninety percent of the publications on this topic don't actually educate their readers and fail to provide an effective means of nourishment. If they did, then most people around the world would be in excellent health and enjoy both a well-built figure and a long life.

Reality would indicate, however, that what these publications offer is a mistake. Even a tried-and-true diet one woman shares with another (the results of which both women can see with their own eyes) is not always what it seems, since it could be that a person rapidly lost weight because of an overactive thyroid or an intestinal parasite, about which neither of them has any idea!

How Did Diet Collection Get Started?

Nearly every fairy tale starts with the standard "Once upon a time," whereas all popular science speakers generally begin their talks with the words: "American scientists" or "The Americans have found ..." So, it would be easy to imagine and make a confident guess that diets had their beginnings in the United States.

The first half of the twentieth century was filled with tragic events on a global scale. These include the First and Second World Wars, the Great Depression, and the rise of two totalitarian systems—fascism and communism—as well as their long-term consequences. Food shortages during this time were keenly felt by all of humanity.

To feed their soldiers during the First World War, the US government created the Food Administration. While developing its plan for distributing regular food supplies to the army, the FA demanded that civilians, mainly women and children, reduce their food consumption. These directives primarily concerned meat and butter.

In those difficult times, they felt this plan was justified and logical and a show of solidarity and loyalty toward those fighting at the far-off front. To minimize the presence of these products in their diet, women and children had to start following well-planned diets. That is, they had to create special dishes designed to meet the body's needs while considering the availability of certain items.

The word *diet*, which comes from the Greek *diaita*, meaning a recommended way of life, entered popular usage and remains there to this day. An entirely new field of knowledge arose that dealt with proper, healthy human nutrition, taking into account the individual's physical condition, age, sex, type of physical activity, work, and state of health.

The situation of women and children at the beginning of the twentieth century forced them to consume more cereal grain products, legumes, and whatever vegetables were available. Proteins and fats were replaced mainly by carbohydrates, which are converted into sugar during digestion. This process led to weight gain among women, despite food shortages.

The following decade saw food become abundant again, but eating small portions and avoiding meat and animal fats remained a clear, typically female behavior. Real ladies ate little meat, since it was considered a food for men.

Once the heavy frames of women during the First World War had faded into oblivion, only to be seen in old photographs, new vistas opened up for the health industry, along with ruthless businesses that pretended to be prohealth but in fact were only concerned with their bottom lines.

During the great agricultural depression, farmers accumulated enormous reserves of wheat, for which there was no market at the time. To support farmers, the government bought up this produce en masse. Fearing that the price of wheat and meat would radically drop, farmers set fire to their grain stores and liquidated their pig and cattle farms.

This happened despite magazine and newspaper reports of widespread hunger, which included photographs of people standing in endless lines for bread and meat at the store. Six million pigs were secretly butchered, and their meat was buried, burned, or thrown into the Mississippi.

Prior to the Second World War, all research into the health problems associated with flour and sugar consumption had been carried out largely in Germany and Austria. Scientists showed that obesity and many health complications resulted from hormonal imbalances caused primarily by consuming flour-based products and sugar. In his 1901 work *The Principles and Practice of Medicine*, William Osler urged readers to "avoid taking too much food, and particularly to reduce the starches and sugars."[37]

The war interrupted this research. The results of European physicians and scientists disappeared, anti-German feeling swept the world, and the only country left with the funds to continue the research was the United States. The 1940s and

---

[37] Chas Mills, "The Truth They Don't Want You to Know," accessed December 19, 2017, https://obesityrecalled.wordpress.com/2012/12/01/the-truth-they-dont-want-you-to-know-chas-mills/.

'50s saw America begin to dictate dietary requirements—and it continues to do so to this day.

Fear of food shortages triggered by the experiences of the First World War and the Great Depression drove the growth of the food industry, which created cheap, preportioned and packaged products that had long shelf lives but were completely devoid of any nutritional value. Meanwhile, the meat-free eating habits of women and children became the basis for a "healthy breakfast" consisting of oatmeal or corn flakes with milk as well as the unimaginable growth of the soy-based food business.

For readers interested in this topic, I recommend Harvey Levenstein's *Revolution at the Table* and *Paradox of Plenty* and Paul Chek's *How to Eat, Move, and Be Healthy.* While reading these books, every so often, I would smile and think back to my childhood in a country cut off from direct contact with the West, a country whose shops were full of empty shelves and where long lines for any good that did appear were the norm.

It reminded me how much I envied my elementary school friend for her sandwiches slathered with sweetened hazelnut cocoa cream, which her dad had brought from the West. I couldn't even begin to imagine the taste of this chocolate spread, and my classmate wasn't willing to share with anyone. I would resentfully unpack my lunch, lovingly prepared by my mother, which consisted of country-style sourdough bread spread with natural, fresh butter and a thick layer of golden Russian caviar. During those school breaks, nobody could convince me of my mother's wisdom.

I also remember that nobody in my elementary or high school class was overweight—besides my cousin, who seemed monstrously obese at the time. He was the exception, however, and suffered from a genetic predisposition to gain weight.

Today, school hallways and playing fields look completely different, although not much time has passed. Obesity is now a widespread problem, and I'm lucky that this new way of eating and these new diet trends came to my homeland many years after the war, that my generation was raised on healthy meat, lard, herbs gathered fresh from the meadows, and vegetables grown in our own gardens, and not on corn flakes and chemically treated lettuce.

Remember

- Everything we eat influences our energy level and our physical, mental, and spiritual state.
- All the cells in our body are programmed to run two related, specific, and essential functions: maintaining optimal health and fitness at all costs and building and reconstructing what has been damaged or weakened.
- There's no one diet or food product that's perfect and recommended for everyone.

CHAPTER 6

A GUIDE TO METABOLIC TYPES

> Every individual organism that has a distinctive
> genetic background has distinctive nutritional needs
> which must be met for optimal well-being.
> —Roger Williams

In 1956, the famous biochemist Roger Williams published
his pioneering and brilliant book *Biochemical Individuality*.[38]
In it, he showed that people have genetically determined and
highly individual dietary requirements.[39]

The results of his long-term studies demonstrated that
there are many differences between the internal organs of
individual people in terms of their size, shape, functioning,
location, condition, and potential. They also showed that our
metabolic processes varied as well and could run at different
rates in different people. This scientist also stated that people
exhibit different characteristics that suggest unequal amounts
of water and oxygen in the blood.

These crucial observations irrefutably prove that our
differences are in fact not just skin deep. Our bodies' internal
functioning and reactions and the nutritional needs that

---

[38] Williams, *Biochemical Individuality*, p. VII.
[39] Wolcott, *Metabolic Typing Diet*, 26.

depend on them all differ. This explains why one person can lose weight quickly by following a given diet, while another may have the exact opposite experience and gain weight.

For thousands of years, the natural, traditional medicines of every ancient civilization (India, Egypt, China, Greece, and Rome) have emphasized the importance of an individualized approach and the necessity of adjusting treatment methods to the specific patient and not to the "case." This viewpoint, passed down from generation to generation, is in line with the thought quoted in this text.

At the turn of the twenty-first century, nutrition and diet became an area of life that ceased to be a biological necessity and began to function more as a *trend and a conversation topic for snobs.*

Well-known celebrities, models, artists, and film and television stars all tell us about their diets, trendy dishes, calorie limits, and so on. Like exhibitionists, they reveal the secrets of their diets on daytime TV shows again and again, sometimes even revealing the part of their bodies they've managed to change. The names of these miracle diets, revolutionary products, and magical supplements in these presentations change as quickly as fashion fads.

Everything is in chaos, constantly in motion! First, the newest thing appears and captures our attention for a moment with an "original collection" of exciting foods and sensational, novel ways for the lucky few who have heard about them to take complete control over their bodies, and then it disappears.

People climb aboard this carousel of absurdities despite themselves, deeply convinced that they should devote themselves to their health. They give in to the arguments of dubious experts, trends, advertising, and sometimes even simple curiosity.

They try out diets, count calories, buy new medicines, and exchange opinions with friends at the office, in cafés, and in hair salons, and the next day, they find on the pages of another colorful magazine another new, miraculous ... Well, you know how it goes! Over the course of the past thirty years, the mass media have heavily promoted several dietary models.

The 1980s

During this decade, we were made to believe that macrobiotics, vitamins, reduced-fat milk, margarine, wheatgrass juice, grains, and plant oils were products any health-conscious person couldn't do without. Meanwhile, consuming red meat, butter, dairy, and alcohol were roundly condemned with an iron consistency.

The 1990s

The wonderful nutritional benefits of fish oils, wine, cruciferous vegetables, green tea, shark cartilage, sea algae, and Chinese herbs were observed. The so-called Paleolithic diet created a sensation, alongside foods containing antioxidants that effectively fought free radicals.

The 2000s

This decade saw a never-ending explosion of diets meant to rejuvenate, aid, protect, prevent, prolong, suppress—in short, it became a sort of nutritional roulette. Each day, we had a choice of diets: high carb, low carb, low protein, high protein, vegetarian, semivegetarian, low calorie, very low calorie, crash, detox, sugar-free, fat-free, low fat, raw food, 40/30/30, vegan, belief based, ketogenic, and so on.

All these fads are accompanied, to a greater or lesser degree, by cogent scientific arguments demonstrating the superiority of one diet over another. With such a proliferation of new information, it's difficult to believe that Confucius, living in the sixth century BCE, shaped the beliefs of the Chinese regarding food and that these beliefs continue to play a part in their daily lives to this day. Some of Confucius's recommendations are

- Eat only at mealtimes.
- Don't eat food if it smells bad or if its color has changed.
- Eat fresh and local; do not eat food out of season.
- Know the origin or source of your food.
- Meat should be eaten in moderation.
- Do not overeat; control in portions promotes longevity.
- You need not limit wine drinking, but do not drink to the point of confusion.
- Hygiene is essential in food preparation.

I won't quote all the principles he developed here. Yet, it is important to note that since they've worked, they should be treated with respect, reverence, and seriousness and should be passed down to subsequent generations—as they have been for 2,600 years!

I would like to recommend using a certain guide that may help you orient yourself within this completely tangled subject. World-renowned nutritional expert William Wolcott, author of *The Metabolic Typing Diet*, recommends eating according to our own nature and avoiding certain cardinal errors. For example, it would be difficult to imagine that a healthy giraffe (an herbivore) would feel fine following a diet for predatory, carnivorous cats and vice versa!

Metabolic typing is the culmination of seventy years of pioneering efforts and discoveries of medical researchers, including physicians, biochemists, physiologists, clinical nutritionists, dentists, and psychologists. Wolcott based *The Metabolic Typing Diet* upon the work of pioneers in the field, chiefly Francis Pottenger, MD; Weston Price, DDS; Royal Lee, DDS; Emmanuel Revici, MD; William Donald Kelley, DDS; George Watson, PhD; and Roger Williams, PhD.

With respect to the *laws of Mother Nature*, Wolcott distinguished three types of food consumers:

I. **The Protein Type** consumes protein found in anything that swims, runs, crawls, or flies and has eyes; this type is characterized by a fast metabolism, in other words, fast oxidizer.

II. **The Carbohydrate Type** eats mainly things without eyes and has a slower metabolism, i.e., slower oxidizer.

III. **The Mixed Type** consumes protein and carbohydrate types of foods and has an average, mixed metabolism, i.e., a mixed oxidizer.

The differences between individual metabolic types are determined by genetic, racial, ethnic, and even geographic factors. It is obvious that the Inuits' metabolism was shaped under different conditions than the Australian Aborigines'.

To help you determine your metabolic type and adjust your diet to it, let's take a closer look at the characteristics of each of Walcott's categories.

The Protein Type (naturally found in Russia, Canada, Tibet, and so on)—this type is primarily composed of people whose genetic makeup was formed in regions of the earth with long, cold winters, which make it impossible to access plant-based foods for a significant part of the year.

The inhabitants of these areas have a daily diet consisting of over 60 percent animal source foods, with the remaining 40 percent being plants. They consume nuts, seeds, root vegetables, berries, fruits, and herbs only when they appear naturally in their environment.

This type of food consumer likes to eat, instinctively realizing that animal protein is the most important raw material for the formation and regeneration of blood cells, muscles, and other tissues and that it provides energy and is necessary to maintain a certain body temperature. The food that could be gathered or grown was not enough to ensure a balance of energy, which in turn could lead to a natural disadvantage in the fight for survival with other creatures cleverer or more specialized in this arena.

So, when representatives of this metabolic type eat according to the rules for other types (a carbohydrate-based or mixed diet), they become depressed, nervous, and fatigued.

When they are hungry, they become irritated, angry, and impatient. Their organism quickly burns off sugars, which is why they have a nearly uncontrollable appetite when faced with a lack of protein or fat. They demonstrate a greater need for the purines (amino acids) found in dark cuts of meat, such as chicken thighs, red meat, caviar, sardines, and anchovies.

Their characteristic behavior includes falling asleep on a full stomach and waking up in a good mood only when they've eaten a meal with an appropriate amount of meat and fat before bed. If this essential requirement is not met (if they eat "something light" or "just a little dessert"), they wake up tired, sluggish, and in need of a strong cup of coffee.

This happens because they burn off carbohydrates at an accelerated pace, which causes low blood sugar, or hypoglycemia. When this process takes place in the middle of the night, they feel hungry, restless, and stressed. In such a state, their body will do anything to bring up their blood sugar levels, which interferes with the production of melatonin (the sleep hormone) and other vital regenerating hormones.

The Carbohydrate Type (naturally found in Hawaii, Indonesia, and Colombia, for example)—people from the equatorial regions of our planet belong to this group.

Plant-based foods dominate their diet, representing over 60 percent of the foods they eat, with the rest being animal products. Due to the specific geographic conditions, the high humidity, sun exposure, and so on of these regions, they enjoy an exceptional wealth of fruits and vegetables that is always available and never runs out.

Water resources guarantee a variety of fish and crustaceans, while other species of animals are also quite common. Consumers belonging to this metabolic type are the opposite of the previous group.

The latter have problems burning off sugar, while this group has issues with digesting protein and fats. They should avoid large, heavy breakfasts and prepare their bodies for a large meal only around lunchtime, when they feel an increase in appetite.

They feel good and function just fine on two meals a day. The fact that they process sugars well doesn't mean they can consume them without consequences and in unlimited amounts.

They have to control their intake of carbohydrates and fast food, despite not noticing any unpleasant effects after eating such foods. Their diet should include lean meat (e.g., chicken breast) and light, lean fish. They shouldn't completely avoid fats, either.

The Mixed Type (naturally present in Italy and Spain, for example)—the two metabolic types presented so far were shaped by diametrically opposed climates. But there are also regions of the earth where these extremes don't appear, where the differences between seasons are much less marked.

In such geographic conditions, dietary customs are different, as finding both animal and plant source foods comes much more easily. People belonging to this metabolic type successfully follow the principle of half and half in their diet, that is, 50 percent plants (phytonutrients) and 50 percent meat.

Their diet is not uniform, however, as it changes according to the time of day or season of the year. Their dietary needs oscillate between those of a protein and carbohydrate metabolism, demonstrating an unusual dependency on their psychological state, hormone balance, physical condition, and external stimuli (particularly climate).

I realize the discussion of the preceding issues is not exhaustive, and perhaps you'd like to learn more. It's necessary to stress again that these facts are just meant to orient you and help you see that there's no one, universal path to a healthy and appropriate dietary strategy that would please everyone.

What I would like to do away with is the established myth of a magical miracle diet that could meet everyone's expectations. For those who would like to learn more about the metabolic types, I recommend William Wolcott's *The Metabolic Typing Diet* and Paul Chek's *How to Eat, Move, and Be Healthy*.

However, try to muster up just a little bit of patience before you go making any sort of changes to your daily diet. Perhaps some of my own personal remarks will help you deal with some of the dilemmas you've faced as well.

It seems to me that I've got the nomadic spirit of a world explorer. Just like Holly from Truman Capote's *Breakfast at Tiffany's*, I've been on the road for years. While searching for interesting people and places, I sometimes arrive somewhere and put down roots for a time.

This means that I not only have to adapt to a new climate and time zone but also learn the local cuisine and find something for myself in it. In countries with four distinct seasons, our metabolism changes depending on whether it's winter, spring, summer, or autumn.

I've noticed that in winter (in Poland or Russia), I eat like a protein type. As such, my meals are made up of about 70 percent meat and animal fats and only 30 percent plants. In the spring, I gradually move closer to the mixed model, as the ratio of animal to plant foods in my diet becomes roughly equal: 50 percent and 50 percent.

I follow the rule that vegetables and fruits must come from local growers and must be in season—*never imported!* Observing how I feel while on vacation in the warmer regions of our planet, I've concluded that I'm definitely not a carbohydrate type. Slavic and Jewish blood flows through my veins, so that sort of diet simply doesn't suit me. I experimented with a carbohydrate type diet for a few months, but my digestive system quickly rebelled.

I had periodic cravings for sweets and coffee, my energy levels fluctuated, I had to go to the bathroom in the middle of the night, and I never felt completely full. When those symptoms turned into headaches, problems concentrating, and an inability to control my annoyance and irritation while menstruating, I said, "Enough! I won't torture myself or my surroundings any longer."

With a sense of relief, I returned to an appropriate diet that was right for my metabolism. I know now that, psychologically and physically, I function best after eating a large, bloody steak or the like, served with various vegetable salads.

I've told you about my personal experiences here to call your attention to how important it is to observe your own body, to read its signals, analyze them, and draw the right conclusions.

Remember

- We can only eat right once we've learned about the foods that we consume each day.
- People have individual nutritional requirements that are determined by their genetics, geography, ethnicity, and culture.
- Learning your own metabolic type will make it easier to develop and establish the principles of your own diet.
- Getting our food products from the natural regions where we live (and in their respective seasons) should be a rule in every individual diet.

CHAPTER 7

PROTEIN: THE ELIXIR OF LIFE!

For some time, I have pondered the proper title for this chapter, which is devoted to animal protein. I tried to settle on one that would emphasize the unique role protein plays in the human organism and its functioning. Remembering that every animal and plant on earth is a life form derived from a common "protein foremother," I decided on the present heading, in which the word *elixir* plays a key role.

This term comes from the Arabic *al-iksir*, meaning essence and "the philosopher's stone." Today, we've forgotten its original meaning, and now it usually refers to a magic potion meant to prolong one's life and deliver youth and beauty.

The futile search for this essence consumed the alchemists of long ago and still keeps contemporary scientists awake at night. And yet, the *essence of life is protein*!

For billions of years, protein has, like a mysterious philosopher's stone—a symbol of the original, shapeless first matter (*prima materia*)—created and protected the genetic codes that are the wondrous blueprints of each form of existence.

I'm referring here to the content encoded in the double helix of DNA, which has determined the material shape of life on earth, including our own. Our instincts naturally command us to reinforce the construction and development of our body through food, which allows us to provide it with the right raw materials and components.

We are a reflection of what we eat, where we live, and what we breathe. We are part of the ancient biosphere in which proteins came into being, survived, and still remain.

The origin of life on earth is one of the most common motifs found in numerous myths and beliefs. It is also a problem that has bothered scientists of various disciplines for thousands of years. One of the ancient Chinese Taoist treatises, *The Book of the Way and Its Virtue*, attributed to Lao Tzu (Laozi), [40] wisely and humbly states, "The nameless was the beginning of heaven and earth."[41]

It is now believed that the mother of all life on earth was a single protein molecule. It could only have formed under very specific conditions, when the cooled sphere of the earth was surrounded by a thick fog that effectively blocked most of the sun's light.

In combination with the biogenic elements found in the remaining sea waters, this created the perfect conditions for processes in which primitive proteins were formed from

---

[40]   Laozi is the mysterious figure to whom the Book of the Way is attributed. There is a debate over whether Laozi was even the name of a real person. Laozi in Chinese simply means "old master," a term that could refer to anyone. Laozi is known as the founder of a school of thought called Daoism, but the term was not coined until several centuries after the Book of the Way was written.

[41]   Lao Tzu, *Tao Te Ching* (The Book of the Way and Its Virtue), Poetry in Translation, accessed January 23, 2017, http://www.poetryintranslation.com/PITBR/Chinese/TaoTeChing.html.

special organic compounds, i.e., amino acids. From that time on, they became a component of every living organism.

The appearance of the first protein particle was thus the most significant point in the origin of life on our planet. Svante August Arrhenius (1859–1927), a Swedish scientist and winner of the Nobel Prize in chemistry, stated that life "flowed down to earth on the rays of the sun."

This was the likely beginning of life itself, and these first proteins would go on to leave their mark in the wealth of simple and complex proteins appearing in all living organisms and forming the basic building blocks of tissue—particularly those of humans and animals. They became absolutely essential to the creation and development of our muscles, tendons, cartilage, internal organs, skin, hair, and nails. After water, they are the second largest component of our bodies!

Enzymes (substances that function as catalysts in biochemical reactions, playing a managerial role) are also highly specialized, important, and indispensable proteins. Other proteins include hormones, the toxins made by our natural bacteria, and antibodies.

All proteins are a combination of twenty-two amino acids, organic compounds that are generally water soluble and easily link together to form large molecules. Our body is unable to produce nine of these amino acids and must obtain them from outside sources, i.e., from food. These are known as the exogenous amino acids, also called EAA (essential amino acids).

Amino acids are the fundamental elements (building blocks) of protein and are colorless, stable solids. Compounds containing a large number of amino acid compounds (polypeptides) are what we call proteins. They are used as raw materials for building and repairing muscle tissue and cellular structures. If our diet is rich in amino acids, our body is usually able to produce the others itself (with the exception of EAAs).

However, when we have a temporary or even momentary deficiency of a single exogenous amino acid, it can affect protein synthesis. This is because amino acids not only serve as the initial materials in this process, but they are also the final products of protein decomposition as a result of digestion.

This process is best illustrated by the following example. Say we have to write a letter to a friend using a twenty-six-letter alphabet but without the two letters *E* and *S*. Of course, this is technically possible, but it is difficult, and the absence of these two letters seriously limits our repertoire of written phrases, not to mention butchering our content and intent.

It is in such constrained circumstances that our body still attempts to carry out its tasks of building, repairing, and growing—that is, circumstances in which it is impossible to combine amino acids in various sequences in order to produce the appropriate protein variations to carry on certain metabolic processes.

In the following list, you will find some more examples of exogenous amino acids, which, when not provided through the food we eat, can disrupt the course of biochemical reactions in our body.

- **Methionine** is an EAA that aids metabolism and helps break down fats. It plays a role in removing heavy metals from the body (chelation) to help protect the liver, kidneys, and bladder. It also maintains proper artery functioning and keeps our skin, hair, and nails healthy. It plays a vital role in muscle growth and energy production. Foods such as nuts, beef, lamb, cheese, turkey, pork, fish, shellfish, soy, eggs, dairy, and beans all contain high amounts of methionine. The bioavailability of methionine is greater in animal foods, especially dairy, making these sources ideal for those wishing to bulk up. Although more research is needed, it seems soy and beans may not be the best sources of methionine.

- **Cysteine** is another amino acid that our bodies are unable to synthesize on their own. Supplied to our bodies by a proper diet, it is responsible for removing toxic chemical compounds and heavy metals from the body and protecting cells from free radicals. It also aids in the removal of excess mucus from the lungs. Frequent colds and a stubborn cough are both signs of a deficiency in this amino acid. Cysteine also fights aging. Shown to be highly effective in ameliorating copper toxicity, it also works to stop the damaging activity of free radicals in smokers and heavy drinkers. And that's not all: the health of your hair, skin, and nails also depends on this amino acid. Finally, cysteine also plays an important role in producing glutathione, a powerful antioxidant. While healthy people can produce enough cysteine from methionine, the essential amino acid that forms the basic building block of cysteine, stress or illness can hinder this ability. That's when a cysteine-rich diet is needed. This means a diet that provides cysteine or the related compound cystine, which exists naturally in many foods. To boost your cysteine intake, the best foods to eat are eggs, cottage cheese, poultry, duck, plain yogurt (not sweetened), ricotta cheese, broccoli, red pepper, and garlic.

Once you learn the biochemical responsibilities of these two amino acids and then imagine that one of them is missing, it's easy to imagine the fatal outcomes and numerous health problems that could result (for example deficiency in methionine can lead to fatty liver and depression). And that's not all!

It is also interesting that amino acids are organic compounds whose molecules contain two functional groups: amines (which are alkaline) and carboxyl groups (which are acidic). Thanks to these functional groups, amino acids help maintain the pH balance of our tissues and blood.

When we have insufficient protein in our diet, our blood tends to become excessively acidic or alkaline depending on the food we've consumed. Protein is essential for our body's correct and consistent development and is also responsible for a stable and healthy endocrine system. It plays a vital role in the lactation process during breastfeeding. It also has an important part in the blood-clotting process.[42]

There are two main types of protein: complete proteins, known as animal proteins, and incomplete proteins, found in plants. Animal fats are widely known to be the only direct, natural source of vitamins A and D (more on fats and

---

[42] Sally Fallon and Mary Enig, *Nourishing Traditions* (Washington: New Trends Publishing, 2007), 26.

vitamins later), but the fact that *only* animal protein provides *all the essential amino acids* may surprise many. So, let's repeat it again: *a complete set of proteins* is present only in animal protein.

Plant protein lacks many of the essential amino acids, which is why it can't be used as the primary source of these acids in our diet. Any missing amino acids should be provided via supplements, and these must be used according to the body's needs at the time. Like the saying goes, "God always forgives, man sometimes forgives, but nature never forgives." Our body *must* ingest *all* essential amino acids (EAAs) in order to produce other proteins from them.

If people think that they'll get around to it someday (when it's a better time), they're in for a big disappointment. After all, one needn't wait long to see the effects.

Brittle bones, nervous system disorders, a decreased sex drive, loss of concentration, insomnia, sensitivity to pain—these are only a few of the many negative results that can occur when we pretend to be cleverer than nature. I've already mentioned that there's no one universal diet, so it is easy to see that the need for amino acids is also highly individualized. It not only depends on our age, sex, job, lifestyle, and living conditions but also our race. Those with darker complexions may have a significantly greater need for tryptophan, which is used to produce serotonin and melatonin, while carnitine deficiencies can appear in people who have experienced long-term muscle fatigue or adrenal fatigue (burnout). This last nutrient, more specifically known as L-carnitine, helps transport fatty acids into the muscles, where they can be used for energy.

Vegetarians, in particular, are at risk for low carnitine levels. The reason is twofold. First, we obtain L-carnitine only from animal-based foods. Second, we need nutrients such as vitamin C, niacin, vitamin B6, iron, and the amino acid L-lysine to synthesize carnitine. Since the mainstays of many vegetarian diets are low in L-lysine,[43] vegetarians may be less able to synthesize carnitine. When grains are cooked or toasted, the L-lysine is destroyed.[44]

These deficiencies can be eliminated by adding mutton, lamb, or beef dishes to your diet. The importance of this decision is illustrated by the fact that almost no plant-source foods contain tryptophan, cysteine, threonine, phenylalanine, or tyrosine.

In our bodies, only tryptophan is responsible for our appetite, sleep quality (hence tryptophan in turkey sometimes being blamed for making people sleepy), and the intensity of our psychological reactions. Symptoms of a tryptophan deficiency may include depression, anxiety, irritability, impatience, impulsiveness, poor concentration, sudden weight loss, slow growth in children and young people, insomnia, overeating, and sudden cravings for carbohydrates or unusual sensitivity to pain.

To avoid these problems, meals should be made with products containing this amino acid. They include red meat, tuna, clams, turkey, nuts, seeds, and legumes, although these last three contain significantly less.

---

[43] High lysine foods include beef, cheese, turkey, chicken, pork, fish, shrimp, shellfish, nuts, seeds, eggs, beans, and lentils. The recommended daily intake for lysine is 30 milligrams per kilogram of body weight, or 13.6 milligrams per pound. A person weighting 70 kilograms (~154 pounds) should consume around 2,100 milligrams of lysine per day.

[44] Dr. Winston Greene, "L-Carnitine," *DC Nutrition*, accessed June 7, 2017, https://www.dcnutrition.com/miscellaneous-nutrients/l-carnitine/.

In addition to the animal proteins found in our food, there are also plant proteins. They are primarily found in legumes and grains. However, it should be stressed that these sources contain substances that restrict their absorption, which I will describe in further detail in later chapters of this book.

A New Look at Ancient Proteins

As we circle the aisles in the grocery store, we wonder what to buy to make sure our meals at home are sensible, healthy, fresh, and appealing. When this problem started to become a global issue, the UN's Food and Agriculture Organization (FAO) set out to answer this question. Once written, it sounded surprisingly clear and simple: *the first rule of a sensible diet is to eat a variety of foods!*

It was a safe and universal response and considered the possible food supplies in every environment and climate. Consuming a variety of foods (without the use of specialist nutritional knowledge) gives us reason enough to believe that the consumer will find the necessary ingredients for his or her body and will even unconsciously consume them in time.

It seems our ancient forebears had always known this. Generations lived on a diet that largely consisted of meat and animal fat, including insects, grubs, amphibians, birds and their eggs, and sometimes large mammals. They added vegetables, fruit, nuts, seeds, some grains, and the leaves of edible plants to this mix.

These varied products ensured that their bodies lacked for nothing. They contain protein, fat, carbohydrates, vitamins, mineral components, fiber, and water. Our ancestors who lived closer to today's Ecuador consumed more plants (phytonutrients), while inhabitants of cooler geographical regions ate significantly more meat.

Studies of their remains show that they had an excellent skeletal structure (as I mentioned at the beginning), a healthy musculature, and perfect teeth.

For over a decade, Dr. Weston Price traveled and studied the living conditions and diets of many primitive tribes from many geographical regions. The results of his thorough, titanic efforts were published in the 1939 bestseller *Nutrition and Physical Degeneration*.

To this day, his research remains the broadest and most complete study to have been carried out on the subject of nutrition. Its scope was broad ethnographically, culturally, and geographically. It included the people living in the Lötschental in Switzerland, Indians, Polynesians, New Zealand's Maori, several African tribes (including the Pygmies), Aborigines, Scots, and so on.[45]

The scholar collected over 15,000 photos, 4,000 slides, and a wealth of films to document his findings.[46] An author of a review in the prestigious Canadian publication *Medical Association Journal* enthusiastically deemed Dr. Weston Price's book a masterpiece of research.

It also expressed admiration for the role the scientist played in exploring the issue of nutrition itself, comparing him to Ivan Pavlov. Admiration of the scholar's work remained high

---

[45] "Nutrition and Dental Caries: A Survey of the Literature of Dental Caries," the National Research Council (US), Committee on Dental Health, National Academy of Sciences, 1952, 429.

[46] *Dental Items of Interest* 70 (1948): 426, accessed via https://en.wikipedia.org/wiki/Weston_Price#cite_note-22.

even many years later: in a 1950 review in the journal *The Laryngoscope*, it was proposed that Dr. Price be called "the Charles Darwin of Nutrition."[47]

The researcher's epic discoveries not only shocked the world of the midtwentieth century but continue to amaze us today. He discovered fourteen populations that enjoyed beautiful, straight teeth free of cavities; were exceptionally immune to disease; and boasted resilient, healthy physiques and an excellent physiology—so long as they followed their traditional diets, which were rich in the most important nutrients.

He demonstrated beyond a doubt the connection between a diet rich in animal fats and robust health and physical fitness.

Just like Price, early explorers noted that the Aborigines were "well formed; their limbs are straight and muscular, their bodies erect; their heads well shaped; the features are generally good; teeth regular, white and sound. They are capable of undergoing considerable fatigue and privations in their wanderings, marching together considerable distances." Other noted attributes included physical dexterity and strong eyesight, which allowed them to spot distant stars or prey that their civilized counterparts were unable to see without technology's help.[48]

Dr. Price also observed that those tribes whose diets were high in legumes or grains, while they were admittedly

---

[47]   I. H. Jones, et al., "Nutrition and the Eye, Ear, Nose and Throat (with Excerpts from the Literature)," *Laryngoscope* 60 (December 1950): 1210–1216.

[48]   Sally Fallon and Mary G. Enig, "Australian Aborigines: Living Off the Fat of the Land," The Weston A. Price Foundation, January 1, 2000, http://www.westonaprice.org/health-topics/australian-aborigines-living-off-the-fat-of-the-land/. See also Arnold de Vries, *Primitive Man and His Food* (Chandler Book Co.: 1952).

healthier than so-called civilized people, demonstrated decidedly weaker teeth and a weaker musculature than tribes whose diets were predominantly fish and meat.[49]

Meat-eating peoples have always been stronger than those who ate more plant-based foods.

It should also be noted that Dr. Price never once found an avowed vegetarian culture during his scientific expeditions.

The anthropological data irrefutably shows that all societies around the world demonstrated a clear preference for animal-based foods and fats and only began to follow a vegetarian diet when forced to do so by exceptional circumstances (e.g., war, enslavement, or natural disasters).

Yet, when the societies being studied began to adopt the eating habits of Westerners and introduced refined flour, sugar, and industrially produced vegetable oils to their diet, they suffered rapid physical degeneration. Health problems appeared *immediately*, while anatomical defects (in particular, narrow jaws and crooked teeth) appeared within the following generations.

As an example, the Pima Indians (*Akimel O'odham*) of Arizona had the highest rate of diabetes of any population in the world in 2006. This was coupled with staggering obesity rates (about 70 percent) and hypertension. Yet things had once been very different. Before their first contact with settlers, the Pima had subsided on beans, corn, and squash, supplemented with wild fish, game, and plants. Like most native people, they had been thin and healthy while on their traditional diet. But settlers placed new demands on natural resources,

---

[49] Sally Fallon and Mary Enig, *Nourishing Traditions* (Washington: New Trends Publishing, 2007), 27.

resulting in famine, and Uncle Sam's attempts to solve the problem with nothing but processed foods and refined flour and sugar soon brought about the situation we have today.[50]

The negative effects are not limited to North America, either. Down in New Zealand, it is reported that one in five Māori children and two in five Māori adults are obese. Māori adults also exhibit higher rates of ischemic heart disease, stroke, diabetes, medicated high blood pressure, chronic pain, and arthritis. Additionally, asthma affects nearly one in five Māori adults and children.[51]

What to do? According to Auckland University of Technology professor of public health Grant Schofield, the Māori should go back to their traditional diet, even though such a diet goes against today's conventional "low-fat" wisdom: "What Māori ate before Pakeha turned up was most likely a diet that was highish in fat, moderate in protein and relatively low in carbohydrate, and that's true across the whole Pacific region. And you can go and study people who are still eating that way, who are more or less disease free."[52]

---

[50] Stephan Guyenet, "Lessons from the Pima Indians," *Whole Health Source*, May 15, 2008, http://wholehealthsource.blogspot.ru/2008/05/lessons-from-pima-indians.html.

[51] "The Health of Maori Adults and Children," New Zealand Ministry of Health, March 22, 2013, http://www.health.govt.nz/publication/health-maori-adults-and-children.

[52] "Pre-European Diet 'Best for Maori,'" Radio New Zealand, November 20, 2013, http://www.radionz.co.nz/news/te-manu-korihi/228291/pre-european-diet-'best-for-maori'.

See also Grant Schofield, "NZ's Health Leaders Respond to Our Research Publicity: Saturated Fat … It's Bad, Low Carb Radical and Unsafe," *Science of Human Potential* blog, October 31, 2013, https://profgrant.com/2013/10/31/nzs-health-leaders-respond-to-our-research-publicity-saturated-fat-its-bad-low-carb-radical-and-unsafe/.

These are the results of giving up a traditional diet, understood as natural, unprocessed foods from wild animals or animals raised on open grazing lands.

Meanwhile, the widespread belief that a high-protein diet leads to a weaker skeletal system (osteoporosis), as well as heart and kidney disease, cancer, and obesity is not confirmed by scientific or anthropological studies. These illnesses are twentieth-century phenomena, while people have been eating meat and animal fats since time immemorial.

There are at least several populations in the world (the Innu, Maasai, Swiss, and Greeks) whose traditional diet is extremely rich in animal products, and yet they do not suffer from the previously mentioned ailments. This proves that it is not animal-based foods that are to blame for these illnesses.

Insufficient protein leads to damage to the cardiac muscles and may be one cause of coronary heart disease.[53] Excessive consumption of protein is also undesirable and potentially unsafe. This is because excess animal protein is digested much more slowly and stays longer in the intestines.

We can easily envision the results if we picture meat left out for a long time at human body temperature: 98.6°F (37°C). Putrefaction sets in, and the rapid growth of various dangerous bacteria begins to threaten our health.

Once they enter the circulatory system, they become a source of many illnesses, e.g., premature arteriosclerosis. The USDA recommends 46 grams (around 1.6 ounces) of protein

---

[53] J. G. Webb et al., *Canadian Medical Association Journal* 135:7 (1986): 753–8. See also Fallon, 2009, 27.

each day for women and 56 grams (around 2 ounces) for men. Some people, e.g., athletes, miners, lumberjacks, and pregnant and breastfeeding women may need more, according to WebMD's recommendations.[54]

Moderation and common sense are the foundations of a healthy and proper diet. As the old folk wisdom goes, the poor and the rich are the ones who eat the worst; the best solution seems to be not too much and not too little.

The Secrets of Protein Cooperation

Few of us know that proteins cannot be properly synthesized without fats and vitamins. These substances form a friendly allied army in the complicated biochemical processes taking place inside our body. So, they can't be overlooked in any sensible, healthy diet.

If these substances have been relegated to the margins of your diet up until now, it's time for a change, since they form an inseparable combination with protein in nature. Eggs, fish, meat, and milk are proof of this.

Only we humans are under the arrogant impression that we know everything better. Perhaps, we sometimes do, but then we cynically take financial advantage of others' ignorance!

A high-protein diet without fat leads to serious health problems and vitamin A and D deficiencies.

---

54   WebMD Medical Reference, "Protein: Are You Getting Enough?", Reviewed by Kathleen Zelman on November 12, 2018, https://www.webmd.com/food-recipes/protein.

Vitamin A

Vitamin A is found primarily in animal products. Plants contain beta-carotene. This provitamin A[55] has much weaker biological effects than the vitamin A found in such products as liver (e.g., beef, chicken, etc.), egg yolks, kidneys, and the livers of saltwater fish. Aware of this, ancient Chinese and Egyptian physicians used chopped, half-raw liver to treat so-called night blindness (nyctalopia) and considered it to be the most effective medicine for many other diseases.

Beta-carotene is *not* identical to vitamin A (retinol). Carotene must first be converted to a form of vitamin A (retinol) that the body can use. The conversion of carotene into vitamin A can only take place in the presence of bile salts. This means that fat must be consumed with carotene, as it stimulates bile production. So, we should drink carrot juice with, for example, olive oil, fresh cream, or butter. Otherwise, we're simply consuming colored sugar water!

Specific enzymes are needed to break down the carotene and convert it to retinol. There are some groups of people who are unable or have a limited ability to convert beta-carotene into vitamin A. They include infants, persons suffering from an underactive thyroid, patients with impaired gallbladder functioning, and diabetics.[56]

Therefore, making plant-based foods your only source of this vitamin is not the best idea. Although the food industry has popularized hardened vegetable oils (margarines, vegetable

---

[55] A provitamin is a substance that may be converted within the body to a vitamin. Provitamin A is beta-carotene.

[56] Enig and Fallon, *Eat Fat Lose Fat*, 54.

butters, and so on) because of their greater ease of use, I definitely recommend farm-fresh butter. It should be present in every diet.

Grass-fed butter is rich in vitamin A and ensures that your intestines get enough of the healthy fats needed to convert plant carotenes into active vitamin A. It may be hard to believe that one piece of our diet can have such a widespread effect on our body: vitamin A facilitates the body's use of protein and minerals, helps the thyroid function properly, participates in the production of renal hormones, ensures calcium absorption, facilitates the assimilation of proteins, supports the endocrine system, and plays a decisive role in the health of our sight and skin. The benefits certainly don't end there, but to list all of them would go beyond the scope of this publication.

Vitamin D

Nearly every tissue and cell in our body has a vitamin D receptor. Vitamin D is essential for a healthy nervous system and proper growth, as well as for mineral metabolism (without enough activated vitamin D in the body, dietary calcium cannot be absorbed), muscle tension, insulin production, and even the reproductive process and functioning of the immune system. Vitamin D_2 (plant form: ergocalciferol) and D_3 (the animal form is vitamin D_3, or cholecalciferol) are not biologically active; they must be modified in the body to have any effect. For this process to happen, cholesterol is needed. We convert cholesterol to 7-dehydrocholesterol, which is a precursor of vitamin D_3. The main sources of vitamin D are fish oil, milk, eggs, and butter—and thus natural animal protein. It is also created from provitamins under the influence of ultraviolet rays, but this is only a secondary source.

When protein is consumed without the fat-soluble nutrients necessary for its absorption and assimilation, many aspects of the body's functioning are disrupted.

From the preceding examples, one can see that protein interacts with other substances in the metabolic process and that their presence is essential for this process to be properly carried out. As such, it is better not to take fat-free protein supplements or consume the low-fat or skim dairy products that line our supermarket's shelves. Furthermore, labels such as 0 percent fat and 0.5 percent fat should be treated as serious warnings not to buy these products, rather than incentives.

I encourage you to eat your crispy chicken skins without any pangs of guilt and not to trim off the fatty parts of your favorite cold cuts. Yes, you can treat yourself to these delicacies, not just because they taste good, but because they're good for you too!

So let the good times roll! Just remember to make sure that the protein, fats, and milk products you consume with such delight come from healthy animals raised in humane conditions, animals that are given access to uncontaminated grasses in open fields and fresh air and exposure to sunlight (vitamin D_3) and are not treated with artificial hormones or antibiotics.

If you're unsure and don't want to go to the trouble to find such foods, it's better to simply get rid of these delicacies before you cook or roast them and thereby avoid the toxins that build up in animal fat. People store toxins in their fat cells too. So be smart when making such a decision: *take a good look at your weaknesses!*

This is one of the greatest challenges a lot of us face in clean, whole eating. You can walk into almost any grocer today and opt for the organic and locally grown fruit and veggies, organic legumes, nuts, seeds, and other plant-based foods. You know then your food is pesticide-free and has been grown without chemical fertilizers, and you could say it was produced humanely as far as plant life is concerned.

When it comes to your animal-based proteins, however, things become more complex. This is because there are more factors that plug into the equation to yield the perfect meat, egg, or dairy protein sources—and a lot of flexibility and varied interpretations when we look at farming terms.

Organic versus Industrial Farming

First, it's important to keep in mind that industrial farming techniques are relatively new. What we think of when we say commercial, conventional, or industrial farming—the use of chemical fertilizers, developed seed varieties, and heavily mechanized methods—only started about midway through the twentieth century.

These methods went on to include the chronic use of hormones and antibiotics and increasingly questionable practices for animal farming at scale, such as the following.

- Overcrowded barns where chickens and hens may spend their entire lives, often in cages.

- Pigs raised in overcrowded warehouses, wading through their own manure.
- Cattle may live outdoors, but they spend most of their time on crowded feedlots without shelter. Practices such as castration, horn removal, and branding are still common.

Before industrial farming, methods were essentially organic, as chemical inputs weren't used. Farms, for the most part, were much smaller than the commercial farms we see today. There wasn't the overcrowding, all the issues of increased risk of disease (and the subsequent increased need for antibiotics), or the sacrificing of animal well-being in order to cut the costs of large-scale production that we often see today.

Organic farming is a more holistic approach to farming. Eating organic protein sources does help to cover some bases of chemical-free, healthy, humane eating. Organic animal farming requires farmers to use organic feed, to not use antibiotics or hormones, and to ensure the animals are raised with relatively humane living conditions.

But there's a catch most consumers don't realize.

The organic farming standards, even more so outside of the European Union, are open to interpretation. You probably assume your grass-fed beef and cage-free organic eggs come from animals that get to move freely outdoors in the sunshine, breathe plenty of fresh air, and experience a reasonable quality of life. Sometimes they do, but it isn't always the case.

The reality is there are certified organic farmers who are raising animals in conditions that are not that much different than what goes on in a factory farm. The sheer number of terms—*organic, pasture-raised, grass-fed, cage-free, free-range*—also makes the discrepancies between industrial and organic even grayer.

It's also important to note that there are nonorganic farms, even industrial, large-scale producers, that practice a hybrid mix of techniques, using fewer chemical inputs and providing healthy living environments for their animals. There are also smaller farms that follow biodynamic, sustainable, organic practices but aren't certified simply because getting certified is expensive for the farmers themselves.

Let's take a deeper look into modern farming practices to help you learn how to source clean, healthy, humane protein.

Unraveling Cage-Free and Free-Range Terminology

Cage-free specifically means that the birds do not live in a cage. That doesn't mean they ever go outdoors, breathe fresh air, soak in the sun, or enjoy fresh growing foliage and buzzing insects around the farm. Hens that live in a barn and never go outside are still defined as cage-free. Even free-range eggs don't always come from happy, content birds, wandering through lush fields as we imagine. Free-range regulations only require the birds to have access to the outdoors.

When you break it down, the terms *cage-free* and *free-range* are misleading. It is a step up from nothing, but unless you know the conditions of the farm you buy your eggs or your chicken from, "better" may be a negligible difference.

Take, for example, the 2016 investigation into a cage-free Costco facility. The investigators found that the birds were actually attacking and cannibalizing each other.[57] In 2017, Snowdale, one of Australia's largest egg producers, was fined over $1 million for falsely claiming free-range status.[58] When it comes to modern animal farming, what we read on the package isn't always what we get.

In Australia, the government just recently passed a law, in 2017, loosening standards for free-range status. This means consumers are left to search for the stricter accreditation schemes like Humane Choice and Free Range Farmers Association, which require more space and more time outside in order for an egg producer to wear their label.

In the European Union, regulations are stricter. Eggs labelled as organic must also be free-range, and the birds must have constant daytime access to vegetation.

Free-range, organic eggs aren't just more ethically sound; they are also more nutritious. Studies have found higher amounts of vitamin D (when the birds are exposed to sunlight), omega-3 fatty acids, vitamin A, and beta-carotene.

This isn't surprising when you think about it. When hens are outside, their diets include a greater variety of vegetation and insects.

You can see the difference yourself. Crack open a commercially farmed egg and an organic, free-range egg from

---

[57] Press Kit, "Costco Investigation Finds Cannibalism at Certified Humane Cage Free Egg Farm," accessed May 7, 2018, https://www.directactioneverywhere.com/press-kit-cannibalism-at-costco/.

[58] Charlotte Hamlyn, "Egg Producer Snowdale Holdings Docked More than $1m after False Free-Range Claims," accessed April 27, 2018, http://www.abc.net.au/news/2017-07-25/egg-producer-snowdale-holdings-fined-over-free-range-claims/8741706.

a trusted producer. You can see the difference in the richer, bright-yellow-orange yolk.

Just keep in mind, color doesn't always mean more health benefits. Some producers include additives, like dried algae, marigold petal meal, and alfalfa meal in the feed to achieve that orange color.

Pasture-Raised, Organic Pork

In factory farms, pigs are raised in large warehouses with unhealthy conditions, like close quarters and manure buildup—creating a toxic environment that can cause the animals to become ill, so they are regularly given antibiotics to prevent disease. For sows, it is extremely unpleasant—they are often kept in metal cages with limited space to prevent movement and are subject to regular breeding via artificial insemination.

These conditions also are horrific for the environment. In the warehouses, factory farmers have to do something about the tons of created waste. In conventional farming, it may be drained into a large lagoon, which then has to be regularly emptied. It's also common, and totally legal, to blast the manure into the air in a sort of manure cannon over the farm's crops.[59] This serves to get rid of the manure and to fertilize the crops—with old, putrid pig manure. This airborne fecal matter then also contaminates the nearby air and water sources and impacts the people living nearby.

---

[59] Rodney Wilson, "Why Pastured Pigs Are Better," accessed April 28, 2018, https://www.hobbyfarms.com/why-pastured-pigs-are-better/.

Pasture-raised, organic pigs, in contrast, have to spend some part of their lives outdoors. As with cage-free and free-range eggs, you want to look for more information to ensure the animals have more than minimal time outdoors and aren't subject to other unhealthy or inhumane conditions. Look for Animal Welfare Approved meats (granted to independently owned family farms that provide plenty of outdoor time and only use antibiotics when recommended by a vet) and Global Animal Partnership Steps 4 to 5 and 5+.

What to Look for in Dairy and Beef

With dairy cows, you want the animals to be grass-fed and pasture-raised, as well as organic. Cows naturally eat grass. However, in the United States, over 80 percent of lactating dairy cows are not kept in pasture to graze on grass and move around freely in the sunshine. They are housed indoors and fed soy, corn, and hay, in order to increase their milk production.

With beef cattle, one of the major problems is the heavy use of antibiotics. The US Centers for Disease Control and Prevention have found that the use of low doses of nontherapeutic antibiotics is partially behind the "emergence of antibiotic-resistant bacteria in food-producing animals."[60] The CDC then goes on to explain that when we consume these foods, guess what. We can develop antibiotic-resistant infections as well. It can also be transmitted through the

---

[60]   Charlotte Furman, "Antibiotic Free Meats: What Are They, and Why Do They Matter?" accessed April 28, 2018, https://www.washington.edu/wholeu/2014/06/02/antibiotic-free-meats/.

water supply and the environment. It is estimated that two million people are infected and 23,000 die each year from antibiotic-resistant bacteria.[61]

Choosing organic, humanely raised, grass-fed meat isn't just about better health; it's about supporting the farmers who are using sustainable, healthy practices, rather than those who are harming not just the animals and our health but the environment we all share.

Look for certified organic beef and other meats—which means chemicals or sewage sludge isn't a part of the food chain, hormones and antibiotics aren't used, and the animals have access to pasture. You also can look for Animal Welfare Approved, as with your pork, and American Grassfed Certified, a certification for beef, bison, goat, lamb, and sheep that means the animals are able to forage and are never confined to a feedlot. Also, they aren't ever treated with antibiotics or hormones.

Biodynamic certification is another level to look for that indicates a high quality of life—and therefore a healthier protein source for you. Established in 1928 and managed by Demeter International, it requires the entire farm to be certified. Animals are treated humanely, and crops and feed are organic. Biodynamic preparations are regularly used and a portion—at least 10 percent—of the farm is designated specifically for biodiversity.

[61] Charlotte Furman, "Antibiotic Free Meats: What Are They, and Why Do They Matter?" accessed April 28, 2018, https://www.washington.edu/wholeu/2014/06/02/antibiotic-free-meats/.

But All These Certifications Raise the Price of Food!

When you look at what is going on in farms all over the globe, how it impacts human health in terms of increased health risks to you and society, the reduced nutritional value, and the environmental impacts, you have to look at value, not price.

You are getting a greater value when you shop for clean, organic, humanely raised protein sources. Not just in that one meal—when you sit down to your free-range, nutrient-packed poached eggs and avocado or your epic steak salad made with biodynamic beef and organic veggies—you're supporting your health, the health of your family, the health of your community, and that of the global community in the long run. Your grocery bill may be five or six dollars more each week, but what about your lifetime health costs—or the burden we all bear in the health and environmental costs to society as a whole?

When you truly weigh the choice—is healthy, clean eating more expensive? Or is there a higher price to pay for purchasing and consuming foods from factory-farmed animals?

The Rumor: Vegetarians Live Longer than Meat Eaters

The average human life span increased enormously in the twentieth and early twenty-first centuries. This was influenced by many factors, the most important of which was the growth of medicine and improved health-care standards. However, while traveling through some regions of our globe, we sometimes come across centenarians for whom all the statistical data on the human life span cease to apply. To give you an idea of the numbers, there are an estimated six hundred supercentenarians in the world (people over the age of 110), while the number of centenarians is likely over 600,000.[62] The United States is home to around 100,000 centenarians, with 40,000 living in Japan and 8,500 in England and Wales. Once we go above 115 years of age, the figures drop to around a dozen worldwide. For reference, the oldest person who ever lived, Jeanne Calment, reached age 122. Later, there was Japan's Misao Okawa, who was named the world's oldest person in 2013 at the age of 114 and who died April 1, 2015, at 117. As for men, the Gerontology Research Group cited Sakari Momoi of Japan as the world's oldest living man at 111, following the death (also at age 111) of Dr. Alexander Imich of New York City in June 2014.[63]

While these are certainly outliers, we've also heard stories for years about certain ethnic groups who are said to enjoy exceptional longevity. Despite researchers' later doubts regarding the authenticity of such information, interest in the lifestyles, diet, and living conditions of these societies remains to this day. This is especially true of the Abkhazians, who live in the Caucasus mountains in northwest Georgia; the inhabitants of the village of Vilcabamba in the Andes of southern Ecuador (Loja Province); and the Hunza people (Hunzakuts) living in the Himalayas of northern Pakistan.

---

[62] "Supercentenarians around the World," *Christian Science Monitor*, August 10, 2010, http://www.csmonitor.com/World/2010/0810/Supercentenarians-around-the-world/.

[63] Tanya Lewis, "World's Oldest Woman Revealed Her Secret to Long Life," LiveScience, April 1, 2015, http://www.livescience.com/50340-worlds-oldest-woman-died.html.

Vegetarians often try to convince others that animal protein is the primary culprit in the shortening of the human life span. It should be emphasized that this conviction is not confirmed by either the anthropological data concerning primitive societies or observations of the peoples mentioned here. While many centenarians live in these mountain areas, none of those encountered so far have completely eliminated animal protein from their diet. Their diets include meat (pork, goat, lamb, and mutton), animal fats, and high-fat, unprocessed milk products (from both cows and goats). They lead an active lifestyle; they perform the work of shepherds, farmers, and craftsmen; travel on foot; and rarely (if ever) use mechanical means of transport.

In addition to researchers' reports, we also have personal anecdotes. The well-known and widely loved Polish humanities professor Aleksey Awdiejew (a Russian-by-descent actor, satirist, and essayist) recalls,

> I've seen with my own eyes several people from the Caucasus who were over a hundred years old and who had eaten fatty, fried lamb their entire lives, washing it down with red wine. My own meat-eating great-grandmother and no less carnivorous grandmother both lived into their nineties, and they only complained about those times in their lives when the People's Republic deprived them of their regular supplies of meat.[64]

---

[64] Aleksey Awdiejew, "O wegetarianizmie" [On vegetarianism], Charaktery No. 5 (52), May 2001, 49.

As for our supercentenarians, Okawa told the *Japan Times* that the key to her longevity was "eating delicious things," such as ramen noodles, beef stew, hashed beef, and rice.[65] Gertrude Baines of Los Angeles lived to 115 on an extremely healthy diet: bacon, chicken, and ice cream.[66] And when Edna Parker of Indiana died at age 115, Governor Mitch Daniels was impressed by her diet of eggs, sausage, bacon, and fried chicken. As he quipped, "I guess we'll have to rethink lard."[67]

In Europe, the greatest longevity can be seen among the Swiss, who live in analogously mountainous regions and follow a similar diet. However, the inhabitants of southern India and Pakistan who follow a vegetarian diet, commonly for economic reasons and sometimes not by choice, are known to have the one of shortest life expectancies (besides the countries affected by the HIV/AIDS plague and some African countries) in the world: sixty-eight years and sixty-six years.[68]

This is due to food scarcity and a lack of animal protein in their diet, among other reasons, such as pollution, high infant mortality, and so on.

---

[65] "World's Oldest Person Misao Okawa Dies at 117," *Japan Times*, April 1, 2015, http://www.japantimes.co.jp/news/2015/04/01/national/worlds-oldest-person-misao-okawa-dies-117/#.WE_KT4RojzJ.

[66] "World's Oldest Person Dies in LA at 115," Associated Press, September 11, 2009, http://www.nbcnews.com/id/32799091/ns/us_news-life/t/worlds-oldest-person-dies-la/#.WRRr7NykJhE.

[67] Elaine Woo, "Edna Parker Dies at 115; Former Teacher Was World's Oldest Person," *Los Angeles Times*, November 28, 2008, http://www.latimes.com/local/obituaries/la-me-parker28-2008nov28-story.html.

[68] The World Life Expectancy Map, accessed June 7, 2017, http://www.worldlifeexpectancy.com/world-life-expectancy-map.

A surprisingly small number of studies on vegetarianism's impact on longevity are cited in the specialist scientific literature.

Dr. Russel Smith, in his impressive work resulting from years of research on heart disease, has pointed out that animal products—even when their consumption among those studied *increased*—contributed to a *decline* in mortality. Such an effect did not appear among vegetarians.

Proteins, as combinations of amino acids and ever-present components of living nature, are extremely varied substances, which is why they provoke so many controversies, conflicting opinions, and mistaken assessments. I don't wish to be an enemy of incomplete proteins, i.e., those that come from plant sources.

I believe that such a negative assessment does not bear out in reality. A well-prepared vegetarian diet may be considered comparable to one containing meat, because the amino acids found in both plants and meat are identical and the need for them can vary from individual to individual. People who don't eat meat, fish, poultry, eggs, or dairy products need to eat a variety of protein-containing foods each day in order to get all the amino acids needed to make new protein.

With the right knowledge, one can effectively manage the products that contain them. Besides meat and eggs, other sources of easily assimilated protein include rice, milk, cheese, soy, tempeh, sea algae (spirulina), quinoa, and natural, organic yogurt.

However, I would like to draw attention to the critical issue of vitamin B_{12}, where its deficiency could lead to serious and possibly fatal pernicious anemia. The myth has spread—unfortunately not only among vegetarians—that this vitamin can be obtained from plant sources: that it is present in brewer's yeast, fermented soy products (tempeh), and algae.

One could simply ignore this mistaken conviction were it not for the fact that a deficiency in this vitamin makes it impossible for red blood cells to transfer oxygen and nutrients to the cells of our body or that it could lead to serious damage to the nervous and digestive systems.

It is also interesting that (in the view of many dieticians) the consumption of plant-based sources of vitamin B_{12} must be accompanied by daily consumption of bacterial supplements. Why? Bacteria belong to the animal world! Vitamin B_{12} is not biologically available in these sources in the same way that niacin is from corn.[69] This means that the human organism is not able to absorb them.

This was shown through studies of the level of B_{12} in the blood of hundreds of people. They demonstrated the same results both before and after eating, including after eating spirulina and tempeh, which stands as indisputable proof of the body's inability to absorb vitamin B_{12} from these sources.[70]

In response to the argument that only meat is a source of this vitamin, vegetarians bring out the big guns: Vitamin B_{12} is produced by special bacteria in the digestive tract, not only in the human body, but in all plant-eating creatures.

They are right. Yet this is no bazooka but a plastic popgun at most, because the vitamin is produced in a form that the body is unable to use. After all, first an internal stimulus must

[69] Byrnes, "Vegetarian Myths," 2000.
[70] James Scheer, *Health Freedom News* (Monrovia, CA: March 1991), 7.

be sent (known as an intrinsic factor)[71] from the stomach for the absorption process to take place in the ileum.

A proper level of HCl (hydrochloric acid) is necessary to activate this intrinsic factor and the absorption of vitamin B_{12}. The best way to stimulate the stomach to produce its juices is through food, particularly protein-rich food. This could be a piece of steak or liver, according to the logical principle that a substance must be delivered before it is distributed. This intrinsic factor also depends on the body's calcium supply, pancreatic enzymes, and upper intestine pH.

The choice between plant protein and animal protein seems to be even more ambiguous when we come across the widely publicized results of studies on the relationship between eating red meat and animal fats and the incidence rate of cancer, particularly colon cancer.

Let's clear up the current knowledge surrounding red meat consumption and cancer risk. After all, food can only be medicine if you know what is and isn't good for you!

In October 2015, twenty-two scientists from all over the world met at the International Agency for Research on Cancer (IARC) in Lyon, France. The purpose of their meeting was to take an honest, thorough, science-based look at the evidence linking the consumption of red meat and processed meat (bacon, salami, sausages, hot dogs, or processed deli or luncheon meats) to cancer.

---

[71] Vitamin B_{12} requires an intrinsic factor from the stomach for proper absorption in the ileum. This intrinsic factor appears through the production of hydrochloric acid, which is stimulated by the consumption of animal protein. Since a bacterial product cannot bond with this intrinsic factor, vitamin B_{12} is not absorbed.

What they found was alarming and something everyone should be aware of: eating processed meats is a sure way to expose your body to carcinogens and raise your risk of colorectal cancer. It's estimated that the lifetime risk of colon cancer is 5 percent. Eating two slices of bacon a day would increase your risk by 18 percent!

Why does this happen? Conventional processed meats are usually cooked with sodium nitrites. These nitrites combine with amines, compounds naturally present in meat, to form N-nitroso compounds, which are known carcinogens. The risk becomes even more pronounced as many conventionally processed meat products also have sugar added to them. In this case, the sugar combines with the protein in the meat to create free radicals, which damage your healthy cells.

Traditionally smoked meats, sausages, and bacon should be brought back to our tables. When meat is prepared without the use of chemical additives, it plays a valuable role in a healthy (and delicious!) diet.

What about red meat—beef, pork, and lamb? There is enough evidence to say red meat "probably" causes cancer. So, should you become a devoted pescatarian or vegetarian? You could, but if you still consume a high-sugar diet or lots of refined carbs, then you certainly wouldn't be eating a diet for cancer prevention. A good friend of mine is a strict vegetarian—and is fighting colon cancer.

The people who were involved in the research used by the IARC scientists not only were regularly eating meat but were also eating other foods linked with chronic disease, like white sugar, margarine, and refined flour. It's also known that in countries where red meat is a substantial part of the diet, yet processed foods aren't widely consumed, colon cancer is virtually nonexistent.

This points to a more complex reality: it's not necessarily meat but rather the compounds found in meat or other foods when they are processed or preserved. This means bacon and pepperoni, as well as white sugar, processed oils like margarine, and any food items with chemical additives, should be crossed off the list. It is also worth pointing out that colon cancer is tied to an excessive level of linoleic acid (an omega-6 fatty acid) in the body.

High-quality, grass-fed beef may not only be safely enjoyed once or twice a week, but it may also even help in the fight against cancer. Beef is rich in protein, iron, and vitamin B_{12}, and it contains an important cancer-fighting, immune-boosting compound: conjugated linoleic acid.

A study of 6,348 women who were diagnosed with breast cancer between 1976 and 2004 and were part of the Nurses' Health Study (NHS) found that women who consumed more protein, especially from animal sources, had a modestly lower risk of recurrence and death resulting from breast cancer.[72] "There's been a concern among patients and their clinicians that eating animal products might be bad for breast cancer," said Dr. Holmes, lead author of the study. "This study provides evidence that patients can be much less worried about that

---

[72]   Michelle D. Holmes et al., "Protein Intake and Breast Cancer Survival in the Nurses' Health Study," *Journal of Clinical Oncology* 35(3) (January 2017): 325–333, http://ascopubs.org/doi/abs/10.1200/JCO.2016.68.3292.

association. Protein consumption does not seem to be bad for these patients, and it might even be good."[73]

So, yes, enjoy your steak salads, veggie and beef stews, and other fantastic, healthy dishes. An ideal single serving of meat, according to the American Heart Association, is two to three ounces (about the size of a bar of soap).

In the case of our two sources of protein, the arguments for and against seem to be without end. I will give a very general overview here of the most important information to consider.

Your support of one of the options will *always be up to you*; I only wish to honestly share the principles of a lifestyle that has worked for me and has brought enormous results to my clients. I believe that making any sort of decision should be done according to Stanisław Jerzy Lec's wise and witty injunction: "One cannot afford to be blind to any point of view." So, let's look through both sides' arguments and counterarguments.

Some vegetarians state that humans have well-developed incisors and wide, flattened molars that are identical to those of herbivores, making it possible to easily grind and crush their food. They also note the similarities in length between human and herbivores' intestines—they are apparently twelve times longer than their torsos, while the ratio of carnivores' intestines to their torsos is only 3:1. This is meant to prove

---

[73] Michelle D. Holmes, "Exploring the Link between High-Protein Diets and Breast Cancer," ASCO Connection, December 19, 2016, https://connection.asco.org/magazine/exclusive-journals-coverage/exploring-link-between-high-protein-diets-and-breast-cancer.

that the human organism is built to consume phytonutrients (plants).

These arguments are cast into doubt by the opinion of François Jacob, who called evolution the *great tinkerer*, a self-proclaimed handyman astonishing us with its unceasing hyperactivity. It is a perfectionist, constantly fixing, adapting, reconstructing, and refining. So, there is much to indicate that humans are beings that *also* consume animal products. This can be seen in the presence of our canine teeth (made for tearing meat) and, above all, by the production of hydrochloric acid (HCl) in the human stomach, which is not seen in strict herbivores. This acid activates enzymes that break down animal protein.

The human pancreas produces a wide range of digestive enzymes that are necessary to metabolize both animal and plant products. Although humans may have longer intestines than beasts of prey, they aren't as long as those found in herbivores. We also don't have the same type of stomach as herbivores, and we (thankfully!) don't regurgitate our food numerous times in order to slowly chew our cud.

As I've written earlier in this publication, not everyone shares the same metabolic type, and not everyone has the same, standard intestinal length. We digest meat in our stomach, while most of the vegetables and fruits we eat are broken down by bacteria in our intestines.

As a detox or "reset" diet, vegetarianism is a good choice. Taking periodic breaks from eating meat and animal fats can have a positive impact on our digestive system. Complete fasting is even required in the practices of many traditional religions and primitive cultures. These are not just spiritual or mystical in nature but also coincide with periods in which access to food is decidedly limited: late winter and early spring.

For our short discussions on vegetarianism, I would like to end with Gary Snyder's remarkable statement about the deeper relationship we have with our food:

> If you think of eating and killing plants or animals to eat, as an unfortunate quirk in the nature of the universe, then you cut yourself off from connecting with the sacramental energy exchange ... which takes place by that sharing of energies, passing it back and forth, which is done by literally eating each other. And that's what communion is. And that's what the shamanist world foresees ... one of the healthiest things about the primitive world-view is that it solved one of the critical problems of life and death. It understands how you relate to your food. You sing to it. You pray to it. Then you enjoy it.[74]

Animal Protein: Fad or Necessity?

Until recently, we could place complete trust in our body's reliable mechanisms for selecting our food, which were shaped over millions of years by precise, logical, and economical evolution. I have in mind not only "cravings" as a signal to supplement something our body is lacking but also all our senses that give us information on the quality of our food.

---

[74] Wharton, *Ten Thousand Years from Eden*, 7.

Today, these natural instruments are fooled by artificial colors, fragrances, hardeners, and substances that even make us addicted to some products, activating an unconscious loyalty program with some of the foods we purchase. We are not properly informed about the true nature of the food we eat. The truth is that our food products are highly chemically treated, making them much less nutritious than our ancestors' foods.

So, what should we do? Only one thing, really: be an educated, demanding, and cognizant consumer who consistently and absolutely demands organic, humane, and ecofriendly *healthy food* from farmers, producers, and retailers and *boycott* any foods that do not meet those requirements.

We must realize that the phrase *the customer is always right* not only holds true in markets around the world, but it gives *us food consumers* the ability to determine the quality of that food. By not buying unhealthy products, we eliminate them not only from the market but, more important, from our tables! We support small, organic farmers who produce organic food that is free of toxins and thus truly healthy.

I've already stressed many times that meat is present in my personal diet and in those I recommend to my clients. I also continue to repeat how exceedingly important it is that these meats and other animal products come from ecofriendly animal breeders.

I respect the philosophy behind the choice made by vegetarians and vegans who state that their diet is healthier. I only wish to note that maintaining our natural metabolic harmony can be done in different ways and take different forms. Placing one's primary emphasis on spiritual existence and conscious separation from the real world has resulted in many religious people (worshipping according to various religions) giving up meat or deciding to live in a state bordering on complete starvation. Nobody questions their decisions, but they seem to be quite controversial and are often perceived as miracles.

Most of us regular folk, however, don't lead a contemplative life and don't have supernatural, godly qualities, and, deriving pleasure from sex, we are baffled by celibates. Our careers, giving birth to and raising children, our activities outside of work, and the daily household hustle and bustle all demand great reserves of strength and nerves of steel.

We need animal products—rich in so many nutrients—to maintain our proper biochemical balance and health. Mormons, for whom ethical problems and moral responsibility toward others and the world are not trivial matters, do not refrain from meat despite their relatively strict rules in all areas of life. The founder of the church, Joseph Smith, stated that a diet without animal products is "not from God." However, in his "Word of Wisdom," Smith wrote that meat should be eaten sparingly, "only in times of winter, or of cold, or famine" and fruit "in the season thereof."

I don't wish to ignore spiritual growth, as I think it is uniquely important, but I also love this earthly life in my real, biological body, with all its advantages and disadvantages. I get all I can out of life, drawing great joy from its riches, and my only experience with the ascetic way of life is from the histories and lives of the saints. I try to be happier, healthier, and more productive by making *simple* changes to my everyday routine and following the old Chinese scholar who preached, "Transformation comes *not* from looking within for a true self, but from creating conditions that produce new possibilities."[75]

The amount of meat in one's daily diet is a very personal matter and depends on the biochemistry of each person's body as well as his or her lifestyle. I absolutely do not question the fact that one can avoid it completely. Some may need more, some less.

However, if its consumption were really as harmful to people as some dieticians claim, humans would have disappeared from the earth thousands of years ago, because we've been cooking, frying, roasting, and smoking it since fire was discovered, as the heat treatment of meat allows it to be stored for much longer than in its raw form.

I should mention here that some researchers believe such high-temperature cooking *might* create compounds that contribute to red meat's carcinogenic risk, but there's not enough proof or enough data to know whether one way of cooking meat (pan frying versus grilling or barbecuing) is healthier than another. Either way, the problem's not with the meat.

The societies Dr. Price studied valued food from animal sources and served it to growing children, pregnant and breastfeeding women, hardworking young adults, and convalescents. No doubt some may remember a time when liver and onions were eaten once a week in family homes and

---

[75]   Michael Puett, Christine Gross-Loh, *The Path: What Chinese Philosophers Can Teach Us about the Good Life* (Simon and Schuster, April 2016), Book Reviews, http://www.ageinista.com/book-reviews-the-path.php.

the cluster of kids lined up for a spoonful of cod liver oil, which had to be taken with a piece of salted bread.

Beef liver is a remarkably beneficial food for our immune system, and it is a revitalizing food in general. Medical research shows that the body's immune function starts to decline by age thirty-five to forty, which makes it increasingly difficult to cope with invaders as we age. Such a rich source of nourishment as beef liver can help fortify and revitalize the body, protecting against age-related vulnerability. One ounce of beef liver contains a massive dose of vitamin A, as well as enough B vitamins to rival a B-complex supplement. It is also one of the most important dietary sources of copper.

The list continues: liver is a great source of other minerals like selenium, phosphorous, and iron; essential fatty acids; and the all-important enzyme CoQ10, an antioxidant that helps your body produce energy and treat many diseases. Liver is also known for boosting energy, although science has not found a specific cause for this superfood's antifatigue properties. I'm all for it, but I also understand those who have a physiological aversion to eating animal organs. For those, I recommend liver extract supplements.

The conclusion to draw from the preceding discussion is that our body undoubtedly requires the numerous, varied, and unique nutrients that are found in animal-based foods. And for those who for various reasons avoid meat in their diets, there are other sources of protein that can provide the right amount of vitamins and micro- and macroelements as well as calories.

Following these diets, however, requires not only quite a few supplements but, most important, knowledge about food and the way the human organism functions and an understanding of physiology. Otherwise, it's easy to fall victim to one's own ignorance and to be taken in by trends or those offering whatever sort of fraud is available.

Prof. Aleksey Awdiejew, quoted earlier, subversively stated that "vegetarianism is a hidden form of cannibalism."[76] How much truth is contained in those words or whether there's any truth to them at all—you can decide for yourself. I consider the issue to be open.

Remember

- Protein is an essential part of a daily diet for both people and animals.
- Amino acids are structural components of protein that play a role in its synthesis and breakdown.
- A deficiency in even one of the amino acids may have severe repercussions for our body's functioning.
- The vast majority of complete proteins are found in animal sources.
- Variety in your daily diet guarantees that your body receives all the essential nutrients for it to function and grow.
- No study has confirmed the existence of even one traditional society that eats exclusively vegetarian foods.
- Vitamins A and D (along with E and K) are fat-soluble and can only be absorbed in such a form.

---

[76] Awdiejew, "O wegetarianizmie" [On Vegetarianism], 49.

- Consuming protein along with fat is in line with our natural biochemical processes.
- When choosing any source of protein, one should pay attention to the quality and amount consumed in order to avoid any life-threatening dietary deficiencies.
- No, that occasional slice of bacon or bratwurst link will not give you cancer.
- To paraphrase Hamlet, To eat or not to eat animal protein; that is the question. I answer, "But, of course, eat it! Bon appetit!"

Protein-Rich, Healthy Foods

I was born and grew up in a small town in West Pomerania. Every Tuesday and Friday, the town came alive at the marketplace, and crowds of people poured out into the streets, off to do their shopping. I was one of those children who loved such days, impatiently waiting for them and holding on tight to my mother's basket (come what may!). My mother and I bravely marched out to amass our *wondrous treasures.*

The fresh fruit, vegetables, cheese, butter, and cream overflowing in the market's makeshift stalls gave off such strong fragrances that I was left slobbering like Pavlov's dogs. To this day, I remember impatiently blending *kogel mogel* (a popular Polish pudding-like dessert) from the bright-orange yolks of farm-fresh eggs. I try at all costs to recreate these flavors of my childhood in my own kitchen.

In those good old days, our mothers and grandmothers did their shopping according to completely different rules. They knew (and were often on a first-name basis with) the suppliers of the products their families needed. Sometimes, these contacts were passed down through the generations, so that they knew the food they bought was flawless.

It is from this period that I take my unusually emotional attachment to stock soup (known affectionately in Poland as *rosołek*), which I always call …

Beloved, Traditional Stock

> Good broth will resurrect the dead.
> —South American proverb

I make it the way it's been made in my family for ages. I buy an entire organic chicken (not lean filets) and use every part of the bird, including the feet, to achieve the true, perfect taste of chicken stock cooked with vegetables (I add them during the last hour) and spices (bay leaves, allspice) for seven to twenty-four hours.[77]

Every little bone and organ must be used! I don't insist on this out of economic necessity or miserliness but because of all the nutritional riches they contain. There are minerals from the bones, gelatin from the cartilage and feet, bone marrow, and healthy fats our bodies easily absorb.

I also make beef stock using a piece of meat with bones and offal in a similar way, though I let it simmer for much longer (up to seventy-two hours). Such stock is a veritable *health boost*. I use it for soups and stews, or simply pour myself a cup and down it with delight.

I blend in the layer of fat, protein, and other substances that develops on the surface and add it back into the rest of the stock. Adding a bit of dry white wine or (unpasteurized) cider vinegar to it releases the calcium, magnesium, and potassium of the bones in the pot. The gelatin that forms is an excellent treatment for intestinal problems, hyperacidity, and inflammation of the colon.

Such a stock has been known for thousands of years (it's called "Jewish penicillin" in many cultures). And it is sometimes treated as a cure-all—and rightly so! It reduces fever, quickly brings convalescents back to health, warms the frozen, and fortifies the exhausted.

---

[77] A detailed recipe with instructions is in the appendix.

As early as the twelfth century, the physician and philosopher Moses Maimonides prescribed it as an effective treatment for colds and asthma.[78] Today, many scientists confirm these experiences, adding one more benefit to the list: broth strengthens the immune system, thus preventing many health problems. We now know that gut health is directly related to immune health. When you have a healthy gut, your body is more resistant to disease. This is why integrating bone broth into your diet is such a powerful way to stay healthy. It is rich in nutrients that heal the gut, reduce inflammation of the gut lining, and strengthen the immune system like collagen, glutamine, glycine, and proline.

It has been an irreplaceable culinary and medical miracle for me as well. I make it twice a week, and I can't remember the last time I had a cold.

Several years ago, I also discovered the benefits of stock made from various types of fish. Proud of their famous *ucha*, Russians have for centuries prized fish stocks, which contain not only numerous health-promoting minerals and fats but also iodine, which is important for the endocrine system and proper thyroid functioning.

Doctor David Brownstein, author of a book on the subject (*Iodine: Why You Need It, Why You Can't Live without It*), estimates that 40 percent of people in the West currently suffer from abnormal thyroid functioning. This is accompanied by various ailments, most commonly fatigue, excessive weight gain or weight loss, hyperactivity, trembling hands, difficulty concentrating, and depression.

---

[78] Enig and Fallon, *Eat Fat Lose Fat*, 95.

That said, there are other, rarer repercussions, such as heart disease and cancer. So it seems it might be worth spending some time making beef, poultry, or fish stock. I personally love Jamie Oliver's recipe for Sicilian fish soup. (He's the best chef in the world!) My family and friends always end up licking their bowls and can't wait until I serve it again.

Eggs

When thinking back to the culinary yummies of my childhood, I can't forget about *kogel mogel* mixed with honey, cocoa, and egg yolks from backyard or farm-raised hens, which are said to be happy, unlike those trapped in cramped cages in factory farms. As a child, I found this dessert exceptionally delicious, and as an adult, I can't imagine home-cooked food that would do away with healthy, organic eggs.

They contain all the necessary nutrients except vitamin C. Egg protein is very high-quality, and the yolks include fatty acids that are necessary for the nervous system to work properly. If the hens are raised outdoors and fed insects and caterpillars, their yolks also contain high amounts of vitamin D and A, as well as the fatty acids mentioned earlier, specifically DHA.

Eggs are a time-honored food, not only for humans but for many other creatures as well. They have always been present in the human diet. The most ancient civilizations prized them for their nutritional value. Eggs hung in Egyptian temples to ensure a bountiful river flood.[79] To this day, they are considered brain food in China, and pregnant women and breastfeeding mothers eat up to ten a day in the hope that their children will be more intelligent.[80]

Many nutrition guides recommend separating the whites from the yolks because of the cholesterol (this terrifying boogeyman that I will discuss later in more depth). There is no logical reason for this, as both vitamin A and fat are needed for the protein from the whites to be absorbed.

The fact is that the yolk is in many ways much more nutritious, and it is also recommended for consumption by adults for its lecithin content, which helps protect against sclerosis.

Whole eggs are an excellent source of choline—an important nutrient that most people don't get enough of. Studies have shown that about 90 percent of people in the United States do not get the recommended amount of choline.[81] Choline has many functions, including helping to build cell membranes and produce signaling molecules in the brain.[82] Thus, the problem for today's egg consumers is not whether to eat them and in what amount but where their eggs come from!

---

[79] Andrew Lawler, "How the Chicken Conquered the World," *Smithsonian Magazine*, April 21, 2018, https://www.smithsonianmag.com/history/how-the-chicken-conquered-the-world-87583657/.

[80] Enig, *Eat Fat Lose Fat*, 81.

[81] Helen H. Jensen et al., "Choline in the Diets of the US Population: NHANES, 2003–2004," *FASEB Journal*, accessed March 21, 2007, www.fasebj.org/cgi/content/meeting_abstract/21/6/LB46-c.

[82] Steven H. Zeisel and Kerry-Ann da Costa, "Choline: An Essential Nutrient for Public Health," *Nutrition Reviews* 67 (11) (2009): 615–623, www.ncbi.nlm.nih.gov/pmc/articles/PMC2782876/.

When hens are raised in their natural environment, their eggs are healthy, with the optimal ratio of omega-3 to omega-6 fatty acids, that is, 1:1 or 1:4. Meanwhile, eggs from commercial farms exhibit undesirable proportions: 1:16 and even 1:30.[83] These latter figures should be alarming, because too much omega-6 in the body is a precursor to health problems down the road, such as cardiovascular disease, type 2 diabetes, obesity, metabolic syndrome, irritable bowel syndrome and inflammatory bowel disease, macular degeneration, rheumatoid arthritis, asthma, cancer, psychiatric disorders, autoimmune diseases, and so on—all inflammatory diseases. So, it is best to get your eggs and poultry from small farmers who raise them in chicken coops near their homes.

Fish

Humanity has long known that eating fish and seafood is good for our health, but until the end of the nineteenth century, they were considered food for the lower classes and the poor. They were eaten during weekly Friday fasts only to avoid suffering from being famished. With time, such religious considerations thus made fish a more common sight on the privileged classes' plates.

Public opinion about these foods also changed dramatically thanks to travelers who readily observed interesting phenomena in the corners of the world they visited. They met many spry, strong, fit yet elderly people among the fishermen in seaside

---

83   Chek, *How to Eat, Move and Be Healthy*, 69.

villages, who even revealed a full set of pearly whites when they smiled.

When spending time in Poland in the seventeenth century, the Frenchman Guillaume Levasseur de Beauplan, architect, cartographer, and military engineer who built defensive strongholds in the country, noted,

> There is a facet of life where the Poles stand head and shoulders above us, and that is fish. They know them quite well, preparing them so wonderfully and giving them such a delectable flavor that they whet the appetites of even those who are already full to bursting. They outdo all other nations in this matter. This is not only my opinion or my taste, but the French and other foreigners whom Poles have entertained think so as well.[84]

Fish are a good source of complete protein and minerals, particularly phosphorus, the B vitamins, and vitamins A and D. Deep-sea fish are also rich in iodine. Above all, I would recommend introducing small, deep-sea, cold-water fish, such as mackerel, herring, anchovies, trout, and sardines, into your diet. They are rich in omega-3 fatty acids, fat-soluble vitamins, and also selenium and magnesium.

With current water pollution levels, large fish are not as healthy as they once were. The bodies of tuna, swordfish,

---

[84] Maria Lemnis and Henryk Vitry, *W staropolskiej kuchni i przy polskim stole* [Old Polish Traditions in the Kitchen and at the Table] (Warsaw: Wydawnictwo Interpress, 1989).

sharks, and others store metals (including mercury) that are unsafe for humans. Methylmercury is a highly toxic substance that accumulates in fish, crustaceans, and the animals that consume them or are fed fishmeal made from them.

They are the primary source of methylmercury poisoning among humans. The level of methylmercury in our food depends on the environment in which the fish and crustaceans lived, what they ate, and how high up they sit on the food chain.

Methylmercury is particularly harmful to the developing nervous system, above all the brain. Mercury has a negative impact on the functioning of the heart, kidneys, lungs, and immune system in people of all ages. Scientists currently warn that small children and pregnant women should absolutely avoid tuna, as it is extremely harmful because of the presence of methylmercury in the fish.[85]

The chemical is associated with mental disability and abnormal functioning of the nervous system. It is better to eat smaller, short-lived fish that have not had the time to absorb too many toxins. One should always avoid fish from industrial-scale fish farms. They are extremely dangerous to your health. Such fish are treated with antibiotics and fed highly processed feed made from food waste or soy.

This also holds true for crabs, whose meat contains significant quantities of PCBs (by-products of chlorination processes) and other dangerous pollutants. Such products

---

[85] John P. Cunha, "Mercury Poisoning Definition and Facts," reviewed on September 12, 2016, http://www.medicinenet.com/mercury_poisoning/article.htm.

should definitely be avoided; consuming them is incredibly dangerous!

As for freshwater fish, the most nutritious are those from natural water sources, from rivers and lakes far from industrial centers and located in high mountain areas. Most of the chemicals and pesticide residues found in fish of questionable origin can be removed by grilling, as the fat in which they have accumulated is released during the cooking process.

A favorite of consumers around the world, caviar (or fish eggs) has many wonderful properties: it is a good source of vitamins A, D, and E; zinc; iodine; DHA; and EPA fatty acids. But, remember, as always, that caviar is only as healthy and nutritious as the fish it came from. In short, it should *never* come from *farm-raised* fish and *never from fish in contaminated water*!

I try very hard to make sure the food on my table is of the highest quality, and I encourage you to do so as well. I do this without feeling put upon or like I'm wasting my time, since I know my health is worth it.

If you ignore this problem today, you'll soon be helping your doctor or pharmacist buy a new Mercedes or go on that fancy Caribbean vacation, and pharmaceutical companies will be adding even more millions to their accounts! And as the Buddhist masters say, our enemies are our best teachers.

Red Meat

A never-ending source of nutrients, red meat plays a very important role in our diet. Unfortunately, most of this meat comes from commercial factory farms, where the animals don't spend their time grazing out in the fields, but languish in their stalls instead. They aren't given a chance to nibble grasses and shrubs at their own pace but are fed an unnatural diet of grain, corn, and soy. This causes them to develop numerous digestive system disorders and many other illnesses.

They live under constant stress and are deprived of even the minimum natural conditions for their species, such as fresh grass and the freedom to move around. Their muscles stagnate, as running, jumping and even freely walking are impossible in their warehouse-like sheds. Their meat is not firm and lean but stringy and covered in layers of fat.

There are constant fears of epidemics on these crowded farms and of widespread losses among the herd. Antibiotics, steroids, and synthetic hormones are administered not only to sick animals but as a preventative measure to healthy ones as well to prevent losses to the farmer. All of this leads to a fatal chain of dependencies: unhealthy creatures unhealthy meat, other unhealthy animal products, an unhealthy society!

It should be noted that commercially bred animals (despite the loud protests of animal rights organizations) are killed in a way that causes an extreme rush of adrenaline, which can have a negative impact on people consuming their meat. Our ancestors did not raise animals in such conditions and on such a large scale, though they did begin to domesticate them relatively early on.

Since time immemorial, people have been trying to come to terms with killing the animals they raise for meat, with religion often playing an important role. As Michael Pollan notes, "The notion that only in modern times have people grown uneasy about killing animals is a flattering conceit.

Taking a life is momentous, and people have been working to justify the slaughter of animals for thousands of years. Religion and especially ritual has played a crucial part in helping us reckon the moral costs."[86]

Of course, I'm far from suggesting that you start killing animals yourself. I simply call on you to continue to fight not only for humane conditions for these animals but also against losing your moral compass, common sense, and reason in this matter. I'm asking you to understand the sacrifice made by the animal and to respect it more.

> As Pollan notes, all is not lost:
> Despite the relentless consolidation of the American meat industry, there has been a revival of small farms where animals still live their "characteristic form of life" ... ranches where cattle still spend their lives on grass, the poultry farms where chickens still go outside and the hog farms where pigs live as they did 50 years ago—in contact with the sun, the earth and the gaze of a farmer.[87]

By looking for the right labels, such as the American Humane Association's "Free Farmed" label, you can become a shopper who supports these small farms and nonindustrially raised animals.

---

[86] Michael Pollan, "An Animal's Place," *New York Times*, November 10, 2002, http://michaelpollan.com/articles-archive/an-animals-place/.
[87] Ibid.

Such support will ensure we have continued access to the highest quality food possible. Each consumer should make every effort to buy meat from organically raised animals and to get their fruits and vegetables from similar sources.

Numerous studies of meats and animal products show that when these products come from grass-fed animals raised in natural fields, they contain high amounts of omega-3 fatty acids and also the powerful fatty acid CLA, an unusually effective substance in the fight against cancerous cells.

This last acid is also exceptionally helpful in reducing the amount of fat in our bodies, while also maintaining proper muscle mass and boosting our metabolism. The natural food for cattle (and other ruminants) is *grass* found in pastures. This food gives both their milk and other products three to five times more CLA than that found in grain-fed animals. In addition, they also

- have a lower fat content
- boast higher amounts of vitamin E (alpha-tocopherol)
- are rich in B vitamins (thiamine and riboflavin)
- have higher amounts of the macroelements calcium, magnesium, and potassium
- are a healthy source of omega-3 and omega-6 fatty acids
- have higher amounts of CLA, which fights cancer cells
- have a higher content of vaccenic acid, which can be transformed into CLA
- have a lower-calorie muscle layer and yield more meat

The arguments presented here speak for themselves, so I won't comment on them. Meat obtained in this way is free of any sort of chemicals, including antibiotics, artificial hormones, and steroids. It offers real nutrition for our body and soul.

By making an effort to find such meat, we show that we care about our own health and take responsibility for ourselves, while also counteracting the damaging activities of big businesses, which aggressively and effectively shut products from smaller farms and humane breeders out of the market. Through such actions, we set off the right sort of chain reaction: buy healthy food, eliminate chemically treated foods, support organic farms, become a healthy consumer, become a healthy society!

Food commerce will cease to be a threat to our health and will start to provide food that can be trusted! After all, habit and convention are not beyond our imagination and ingenuity; we can start to advocate for our own interests, break the previous rules of the market, boycott the chemicalization of the food industry, and buy only organic food for ourselves! The health and happiness of humankind starts with each of us!

Not only can we affect change with our wallets, but we can also make a difference by acknowledging and speaking out about the hidden price of our cheap, industrially produced meat. As Pollan observes, if people really knew what industrial animal farming in America (now almost all over the world) involved—the brutal, inhumane slaughter of animals raised in appalling conditions—these practices would disappear. So, let's give these animals' sacrifice the respect it deserves; a slight hike in our grocery bill is but a small price to pay. Let's sum up our discussion with Leo Tolstoy's dictum: "God gave food to people, and the devil gave cooks." I believe if the great writer had lived to see our times, he would have accepted this updated version: "God gave food to people, and the devil gave us greedy producers and retailers."

But to avoid ending this discussion on such a cynical note, I suggest taking the advice known for centuries in the Middle East: "What is the medicine for a man overcome by melancholy? Red meat roasted over coals and spiced wine!"

Poultry

A high-quality, lean protein source, poultry plays a starring role in a healthy, balanced diet. It's rich in B vitamins and key minerals like zinc, iron, and copper, and it's an excellent source of highly digestible protein, giving the body the building blocks it needs for growth and repair, sustainable energy, and overall well-being.

Ranging from soul-nourishing chicken soup to roasted duck, turkey, goose, and quail, poultry includes all domesticated birds that are kept for their meat, as well as their eggs. Consumed worldwide, poultry, especially chicken, has become a food staple in many cultures. Its mild taste and chewy texture make it perfect for enriching flavorful dishes with a healthy, nourishing protein.

Poultry has become a culinary centerpiece all over the world, from the Caribbean's hearty chicken and root veggie soup, sancocho, to India's chicken curry dishes and classic French roast turkey with rosemary, sage, and thyme. When you think about the fact that humans domesticated poultry thousands of years ago for food, it's no surprise we have so many delectable masterpieces that feature poultry today.

The exact transition from hunting wild fowl to keeping and raising birds isn't totally clear, but scholars agree it happened about eight thousand years ago in Asia. Humans started raising the wild red jungle fowl—the cousin of the tame, less-social chickens of today. The red jungle fowl still roam around in the bamboo forests of Southeast Asia and India.

From China and Southeast Asia, chickens were introduced to the Middle East, Africa, and later continental Europe via present-day Spain. The Spanish conquistadors may have brought them to the Americas, although there is evidence of pre-Columbian poultry in South America.

Chickens are still sacred in some cultures, being seen as a symbol of fertility, with the rooster being a beacon of virility. In Zoroastrianism, the rooster is viewed as a benign spirit who crows at daybreak to announce the turning point in the endless cosmic struggle between light and darkness.

Health Benefits of Chicken

When you look at how nourishing chicken is, you can see why it has ended up playing such a prominent role in diets around the globe.

Some of the benefits of chicken include the following:

- It is a good source of vitamin D and helps with calcium absorption for stronger bones and teeth.

- The B vitamins in chicken promote immune health, boost energy levels, and stabilize mood by helping the body produce serotonin.
- Chicken is a great source of easy-to-absorb iron, which helps with everything from maintaining muscle health and cognitive function to preventing fatigue and hair loss.
- Copper and zinc strengthen the immune system.
- Selenium is an important antioxidant that helps to reduce the risk of chronic illnesses.

With all types of poultry, when you eat the whole bird, you get both the white and dark meat. The breasts have all the white meat, while the thighs contain the dark meat.

You may have heard that it's better to just eat breast meat. It is, after all, leaner. Chicken breasts are also higher in the amino acid tryptophan, a nutrient you want to get plenty of because it is a precursor to serotonin.

But chicken thighs and dark meat from poultry in general have a lot of nutritional value too. Dark meat is a good source of healthy monounsaturated fats, which are good for promoting weight loss and reducing your risk of heart disease and cancer. Dark meat is also higher in iron, zinc, selenium, the vitamins A and K, and the B complex vitamins.

Eating both white and dark meat will offer the best health benefits. The key to lowering the fat content isn't to leave out the richer dark meat, but rather, to use healthy cooking methods like roasting chicken and cooking it in stews and soups, rather than frying it.

Safe Habits for Poultry in the Kitchen

When preparing any type of raw poultry, it's important to always handle the bird properly. You want to make sure you keep surfaces clean after handling uncooked poultry. Unlike other protein sources, like beef and tuna, this is one meat you don't want to eat raw or undercooked. It not only will have an unpalatable texture, undercooked chicken can be a food-poisoning risk because of the bacteria present on the meat.

Poultry should always be cooked through. You want the meat to reach at least 165° F or 73° C to kill all the bacteria. You can stick a thermometer in the thickest part of the meat to verify the temperature.

If you aren't cooking your poultry within a day or two after purchasing, you should freeze the meat until you are ready to thaw it out and cook it.

Don't rinse raw poultry in water before cooking. This doesn't get rid of any bacteria. After handling, wash your hands, prep surfaces, and utensils with soap and warm water for twenty seconds, at least. And don't let other food come into contact with any surfaces you haven't cleaned yet.

Beyond Organic Chicken

To get all the health benefits of poultry, without all the downsides of commercial food production, choose your chicken wisely.

With organic chicken, the birds have been fed food that's pesticide-free. They haven't been given antibiotics, and they have access to the outdoors. But where a lot of consumers get confused is they assume organic chicken is pasture-raised and ethically raised. As I already mentioned in previous chapters, organic labeling doesn't ensure your chicken lived in the fresh air and grew up with nature's abundance for its diet. Producers only have to allow access to the outside. This means organic chickens can still spend their days in overcrowded warehouses. It's just they are eating certified organic grain instead of nonorganic grains.

For ethically raised birds, look for small, local farmers whose chickens spend most of their time outdoors. You can also talk to your local butcher to see if they source pasture-raised birds.

Another option is to look for trusted food industry certifications like Global Animal Partnership, Certified Humane, and Animal Welfare Approved (AWA). Just as with eggs from pasture-raised hens, your poultry will have access to a better quality of food (nature's table of foliage and insects), as well as the sunshine to increase the birds' vitamin D levels.

Genuinely pasture-raised birds are more expensive, but you are supporting the dedicated producers who are keeping sustainable food production alive while at the same time benefiting your health.

Remember

- Our menu should always be a source of health, pleasure, and spontaneous joy.
- Preparing and enjoying meals should be a time for reflection, psychological processing of the

day's experiences and maintaining interpersonal relationships, not just to satisfy our hunger.

- Proper, healthy nourishment requires knowledge, creativity, responsibility, and an honest desire to achieve it.
- By boycotting chemically treated miracle foods, we demand higher quality from food producers and put greedy poison hawkers out of business.
- Be sure to round out your plate with plenty of veggies and other nutrient-rich foods and vary your sources of protein by including fish and poultry too.

CHAPTER 8

FAT: THAT TERRIFYING BOOGEYMAN

It's harder to crack a prejudice than an atom.
—Albert Einstein

It seems nothing can make you feel so powerless as fighting against stereotypes and those aspects of reality that originally came about as temporary, provisional solutions. The former have been present in the social consciousness for such a long time and have become so ingrained that nobody goes to the effort to verify these oversimplified and often false convictions. Meanwhile, the latter eventually go from being temporary to daily necessities.

This thought first came to me when I began writing this chapter on fats. I recalled my close friend's wedding reception, where, because of the large number of foreign guests, they decided to have not only a long banquet table for all the guests but also several other tables with national buffets, so that those from other countries wouldn't go hungry.

To introduce outsiders to Polish cuisine, our national buffet included *bigos*, rustic bread, dill pickles, tripe, steak tartare, and—most important—clay pots brimming with homemade lard with pork scratchings, onion, marjoram, and caraway. When a long line formed at this display of food, I didn't think everybody was waiting for a piece of fresh bread thickly slathered with lard. The overheard conversations in the queue revealed gluttonous desire, ignorance, and expressions of guilt: "It's so unhealthy"; "It clogs your arteries"; "It's a strain on your liver"; "It's bad for your heart"; and so on.

By the end of the party, some of the exotic delicacies at the other smorgasbords remained practically untouched, while not a trace was left of the aromatic lard on the Polish table. If it hadn't been for the exceptional circumstances and the fact that the whole thing had been a genuine surprise arranged by our hosts, I would have happily prepared a sign for the table's huge awning that would have read, "The idea that saturated fats cause heart disease is completely wrong."[88]

This last sentence is a partial quotation by Dr. Mary Enig, who took up the fight against negative views of saturated fats, armed with incontrovertible scientific evidence to the contrary. I will cite her in full here, so you can appreciate the full significance of the problem:

> The idea that saturated fats cause heart disease is completely wrong, but the statement has been "published" so many times over the last three or more decades that it is very difficult to convince people otherwise, unless they are willing to take the time to read and learn what all the economic and political factors were that produced the anti-saturated fat agenda.[89]

---

[88] Uffe Ravnskov, "The Many Critical Scientists," December 27, 2015, http://www.ravnskov.nu/myth7.htm.

[89] Ibid.

I hope to motivate and inspire you to counter these myths and be unafraid to challenge such stereotypes and undermine their secure position in our lives.

Truth and Myths

> And the truth, before it is revealed to all, face to face, we see in fragments (alas, how illegible) in the error of the world, so we must spell out its faithful signals even when they seem obscure to us and as if amalgamated with a will wholly bent on evil.
> —Umberto Eco

Knowledge unmasks the illusions long held as natural by society, exposing their artificial nature. It shows us that our previous image of reality is in fact not true, radically transforming our assessment of it. This leads not only to the joyful discovery of the truth but also to the more bitter realization that such false certainties have deceived us for so long. For some, confronting clear evidence and real arguments comes with difficulty, while others simply stick to their guns and flat out refuse to bend. In such cases, one can only throw up one's hands and carry on investigating the truth for the good of humanity.

This is also true in the case of fats. The common admonitions to follow a low-fat diet are in fact completely unjustified, even in the most "trustworthy" studies carried out by recognized scientific authorities. Consuming healthy, organically produced animal and vegetable fats supports the functioning of all our body's systems.

Fat isn't merely a source of energy but also an essential building block for our cell membranes and a whole host of hormones and hormonal substances. The energy from fat is generated much more efficiently and lasts longer than that of carbohydrates. Fats slow down the absorption of nutrients and sugar into the bloodstream, so we don't feel hungry.

They also function as carriers of fat-soluble vitamins A, D, E, and K and help convert beta carotene into vitamin A. Many scientific medical publications describe the essential roles played by saturated/animal fats, such as strengthening the immune system, maintaining healthy bones, providing potent energy, ensuring the integrity and proper structure of cells, protecting the liver from harmful substances, and fortifying the body in general. The literature emphasizes the role of stearic acid, found in beef tallow and butter, in lowering cholesterol, as well as its other benefits for the heart. Animal/saturated fats are stable, stay fresh for a long time, don't go rancid easily, don't deplete the body's antioxidant reserves, are not carcinogenic, and do not irritate artery walls.

I am aware that the information presented here may be met with distrust, disbelief, irritation, and even hostility. Yet, I ask for your patience and willingness to learn more about this misconception.

We should learn to differentiate between healthy and unhealthy fats and sort out illusory opinions and conventional wisdom in order to free ourselves from them. Our species' evolution and the gradual appearance of hunting and farming alongside the most ancient gathering culture clearly show that animal fats have not destroyed humankind but have allowed us to survive in even the most difficult living conditions.

So how did conventional wisdom come to place a low-fat diet on such a pedestal? First, dietary norms are *not* built upon sound nutritional science and are *not* set by specialists, doctors, or dieticians but by politicians.

Secondly, the owners of large food enterprises are, by and large, also the owners of pharmaceutical and chemical companies.

Thirdly, as Hitler's right-hand man and the Third Reich's minister of propaganda and education Joseph Goebbels cynically noted, "If you tell a lie big enough and keep repeating it, people will eventually come to believe it."[90] The power of gossip, myths, and stereotypes these days confirms this observation, especially since the mass media eagerly spread them.

If such information is accompanied by alleged studies conducted by alleged experts and topped off with magical figures, then society accepts it all as incontrovertible truth. After all, "when lying judges become many, false witnesses become many." At the turn of the twentieth century, 90 percent of scientific research was funded by universities and 10 percent by pharmaceutical companies. Today, those figures have reversed: 90 percent of studies come from pharmaceutical companies and 10 percent from academic centers.[91] It should be noted that as little as fifty years ago, the pharmaceutical industry still devoted significant sums to specialist-performed research, while today that money is spent on advertising and marketing.

---

[90] Ironically, while this quote is often attributed to Goebbels, he likely never said it.

[91] De Leth, *Oersterk*, 82.

And although "false witnesses are contemptible even to those who hire them," it turns out that the prospect of easy profit often comes before dignity and a sense of responsibility. The April 11, 2012, issue of the Dutch medical journal *Medisch Contact*[92] reports that statistically one in seven physicians has witnessed fabricated scientific results. Nearly a quarter of physicians attested to witnessing the use and publication of only those experimental results that were most favorable to both researchers and those funding the research: businesses.

Unfortunately, the medical, pharmaceutical, and food-processing industries, along with commerce, have created a web of business dependencies that is so precisely organized and has such large amounts of money at its disposal that it not only controls local markets but has undeniably long been a global force.

These ties can be compared to an unhappy marriage of convenience. The medical establishment dreams of new possibilities for treating patients and relieving their suffering, while the business side of the coin wants to continue raking in profits, which would be impossible without the medicinal establishment. Divorce is out of the question!

This pathological relationship has been vividly described by Dr. Denis Burkitt, MD, who received some of the highest distinctions given in the field of medicine in the United States and Canada for his disinterested and forthright work. As he wrote,

---

[92] Joost Visser, "Veel artsen weten van wetenschapsfraude," Medisch Contact, last updated April 11, 2012, https://www.medischcontact.nl/nieuws/laatste-nieuws/artikel/veel-artsen-weten-van-wetenschapsfraude.htm.

Western doctors are like poor plumbers. They treat a splashing tube by cleaning up the water. These plumbers are extremely apt at drying up the water, constantly inventing new, expensive, and refined methods of drying up water. Somebody should teach them how to close the tap.[93]

Being healthy seems to be the most sensible course, albeit not a very lucrative one. This observation may be shocking, but it shouldn't lead us to believe we have no influence here, because *we do*!

Behind the Lipid Hypothesis

Before I present the topic suggested by this chapter's title, let me mention a few facts from the past. These references don't go all the way back to prehistorical times but rather to a reality a bit closer to ours, tied to Polish cultural traditions and culinary customs that may illustrate some of the phenomena that interest us.

Historical sources indicate that the medieval pantries of well-off peasants and most of the nobility were stocked with a wide variety of foods. Alongside dried and pickled fare, as well as fruits and vegetables stored in sand in chests, one could also find salted and smoked beef, game, and pork. The sausages, slices of pork fat, clay pots with sour cream and butter, cheeses, and eggs gathered in their kitchen cupboards

[93] "Sunbeams," *Sun*, January 2016, http://thesunmagazine.org/issues/481/sunbeams.

testified not only to the owners' affluence but above all to their daily diet, which has lasted for centuries and is still followed by Poles today.

The German journalist and traveler Fritz Wernick (1823–1891) was so taken by this diet that he devoted several thoughts to it in his enormous work *Stadtebilder*. Without a doubt, the man was a connoisseur of good food and easily recognized the primary characteristics of Polish cuisine. Here are a few of his observations:

- "Warsaw cuisine has products of excellent quality at its disposal. They are skillfully transformed into exquisite dishes. The food is at the same time extremely concentrated and rich."[94]
- "The nourishing meat of Polish oxen is eaten in considerable quantities here and is inexpensive."[95]
- "Fats, strong seasonings and onion are widely used in Polish cuisine."[96]
- "One can expect to receive healthy and delicious meat dishes everywhere."[97]
- "It is only in Poland that fat, choice turkeys have such an exquisite, unique taste, especially because they do not skimp on butter when roasting, making the meat tender and moist."[98]

[94] Lemnis and Vitry, *Old Polish Traditions in the Kitchen and at the Table*, 267–268.
[95] Lemnis and Vitry, *Old Polish Traditions in the Kitchen and at the Table*, 268.
[96] Lemnis and Vitry, *Old Polish Traditions in the Kitchen and at the Table*, 269.
[97] Lemnis and Vitry, *Old Polish Traditions in the Kitchen and at the Table*, 270.
[98] Lemnis and Vitry, *Old Polish Traditions in the Kitchen and at the Table*, 270.

I should also cite one last opinion from this nineteenth-century foreign tourist, which may come as a shock to visitors of today's Warsaw: "However, one thing common to all levels of Polish society is the complete *lack of obesity*. Among thousands of residents, I never once encountered *a single overweight person* in Warsaw, which is even more peculiar since they eat such rich and hearty food here."

The information and quotations I've cited here come from Maria Lemnis and Henryk Vitry's fascinating book *Old Polish Traditions in the Kitchen and at the Table,* which has been printed in four languages (English, German, Russian, and Polish) and has attracted the interest of foodies and dietary specialists alike.

You've surely noticed the predominance of meat and animal fats in these interesting notes on Polish food culture, and yet the nation survived centuries of various tragedies on such a diet. So, how did heart disease, atherosclerosis, and obesity, unknown to us for centuries, become serious and concerning problems in the twentieth and early twenty-first centuries?

While searching for the causes of heart disease, atherosclerosis, and obesity, which have become commonplace in Europe and America, in the early 1950s, scientists of various disciplines concentrated on the so-called "lipid hypothesis." This term was created and popularized by the researcher Ancel Keys, who suggested there was a strong link between these diseases and animal fat. An American psychologist with a keen interest in nutrition, Keys had been part of many US government dietary projects, including the development of the K ration, a nutrient-rich bar used to feed American troops.

He developed a theory that cardiovascular disease was caused by saturated fat.

Although the "lipid hypothesis" was never confirmed by any reliable scientific research, and numerous errors were found in the experiments that were conducted, Keys still managed to foster acceptance of his theory as absolute truth! The scholar was known for his powers of persuasion, eloquence, and talent for self-promotion. Keys became a national hero and soon landed on the front cover of *Time* magazine.

He and his theory quickly found themselves within the sphere of interest of vegetable oil and food producers, and the "lipid hypothesis" began to receive large financial backing from these circles.

However, several years later, in 1956, Keys suggested that the widespread use of hydrogenated vegetable oils may lead to coronary heart disease (CHD),[99] but, by then, the massive marketing machine that had begun to tout its healthy properties could no longer be stopped. This machine was driven not only by the far-reaching influence of producers but above all by large amounts of money. Keys' publication was passed over in silence, and hydrogenated oils conquered even more branches of the food industry, new sales markets, restaurant chains, and so on.

In 1920, the young, promising internist Paul Dudley White presented to his colleagues at Harvard the latest German diagnostic invention: the electrocardiograph. The machine

---

[99] Keys, A., "Diet and Development of Coronary Heart Disease," *J. Chron. Dis.* 4 no. 4(1956):364–380; op.cit. Mary Enig and Sally Fallon, "The Oiling of America."

failed to arouse any interest in the medical community.[100] It was thought it wouldn't bring in any money because of the rarity of patients with heart ailments, including obstructed arteries, at the time.

Yet, by the 1950s, Paul Dudley White was a well-known and respected internist, cardiologist, and authority in medical circles. He then observed the number of patients with heart disease had increased dramatically from the moment consumption of liquid vegetable oils rose alongside the restricted consumption of eggs, traditional butter, and lard. During a press conference, Dr. White stated, "I began my practice as a cardiologist in 1921 and I never saw an MI [heart attack] patient until 1928. Back in the MI-free days before 1920, the fats were butter and lard, and I think we'd all benefit from the kind of diet we had at a time when no one had ever heard the term 'corn oil.'"[101]

An analysis of the food trade and old cookbooks (like what I did with Polish culinary traditions) shows that as late as 1900, between 35 and 40 percent of calories in the American diet came from fats, primarily butter, cream, whole milk, and eggs.[102] Salad dressings and sauces were usually made from yolks or cream, while olive oil was used only sporadically, not to mention corn or soybean oils. Lard and tallow were

[100] Enig Fallon, "The Skinny on Fats," accessed April 12, 2016, https://www.westonaprice.org/health-topics/know-your-fats/the-skinny-on-fats/.

[101] Mary Enig and Sally Fallon, "Secrets of the Edible Oil Industry (Part I)," Mercola.com, accessed June 7, 2017, http://articles.mercola.com/sites/articles/archive/2001/08/01/oil-part-one.aspx.

[102] Fallon Enig, "The Oiling of America—Weston A. Price Foundation," accessed May 27, 2016, https://pdfs.semanticscholar.org/c929/ad22d48819170127597d26a5e70c38a49021.pdf.

used for frying, while cheeses and meats of various kinds were often served. Just like in Poland, saturated fats had been present in the American diet for centuries, but heart disease and cancer were rare.

Meanwhile, the process of hardening vegetable oils was developed by chemists in 1912, but it was only after World War II that global producers began to hydrogenate liquid oils on a large scale.

Such fats began to be widely used for frying foods, baking cakes, and as a spread on baked goods, while lard and coconut oil fell by the wayside. People began to consume artificial fats in unprecedented numbers—fats which had never existed in the history of humankind.

Methods of extracting fats from plants were also perfected to produce them quickly and in large amounts. This led to a dramatic rise in soy production, which grew to seventy million tons in 1970, surpassing even that of corn. Soybean oil currently dominates the global market, making up 80 percent of all hydrogenated oils.[103] In the twentieth century, the contribution of animal fats in our diet fell from 50 to 20 percent, while in 2009, they represented less than 16 percent of fats used, showing that vegetable fats have become increasingly popular.[104]

[103] Mary Enig and Sally Fallon, "The Oiling of America" (PDF), accessed June 7, 2017, http://www.spiritofhealthkc.com/wp/wp-content/uploads/2014/03/The-Oiling-of-America.pdf.

[104] "Vegetable Oils in Food Technology: Composition, Properties and Uses," 2nd ed. (PDF), accessed June 7, 2017, https://www.researchgate.net/publication/228033593.

Since 1970, the "lipid hypothesis" has become a universal explanation for heart disease, supported by medical experts and by government agencies.

Large amounts of money and pressure surely came from even more effective lobbyists, who were undoubtedly the owners of food processing and production enterprises, as well as pharmaceutical and chemical companies. This cynical plan to eliminate fat and animal products and replace them with vegetable oils and margarine, in combination with the production of medications to lower cholesterol and eliminate all types of heart disease, seems to have been implemented with extraordinary speed and precision.

Yet, the irony is that currently

- About 630,000 people die of heart disease in the United States every year—that's one in every four deaths.[105]
- Heart disease kills more people each year than AIDS and all cancers combined.[106]
- By the year 2020, heart disease will have become the primary cause of death worldwide.[107]
- About 720,000 Americans suffer heart attacks each year; 515,000 of these cases are first-time attacks, while

---

[105]   Centers for Disease Control and Prevention, National Center for Health Statistics. Multiple Cause of Death 1999–2015 on CDC WONDER Online Database, released December 2016. Data are from the Multiple Cause of Death Files, 1999–2015, as compiled from data provided by the fifty-seven vital statistics jurisdictions through the Vital Statistics Cooperative Program, accessed April 23, 2018, https://www.cdc.gov/heartdisease/facts.htm.

[106]   "Heart Disease: Scope and Impact," The Heart Foundation, http://www.theheartfoundation.org/heart-disease-facts/heart-disease-statistics/.

[107]   Ibid.

205,000 happen to those who have already had a heart attack.[108]

- Around eighty million Americans suffer from one or more types of heart disease.[109]
- Cardiovascular disease costs the United States $108.9 billion annually.[110]
- The direct costs of cardiovascular disease in the United States are expected to triple over the next twenty years, reaching $818 billion.[111]
- Cardiovascular disease costs the European Union nearly €196 billion per year.[112]
- Cardiovascular disease is the cause of 47 percent of all deaths in Europe and 40 percent in the EU.[113]

When faced with such dire figures, one might recall the wise old saying "No misfortune comes to a man which does not profit somebody." Of course, we would be wrong to believe that this hypocritical practice does not have its detractors, who are trying to put a stop to it and fight back with their own arguments. Aseem Malhotra, an interventional cardiology specialist registrar at Croydon University Hospital in London,

---

[108] Alan S. Go et al., "Heart Disease and Stroke Statistics—2014 Update: Report from the American Heart Association," *Circulation* (2013): 128, https://doi.org/10.1161/01.cir.0000441139.02102.80.

[109] "Heart Disease: Scope and Impact."

[110] Paul A. Heidenreich et al., "Forecasting the Future of Cardiovascular Disease in the United States: A Policy Statement from the American Heart Association," *Circulation* 123 (2011): 933–44, https://doi.org/10.1161/CIR.0b013e31820a55f5.

[111] "Heart Disease: Scope and Impact."

[112] "2012 European Cardiovascular Disease Statistics," *European Society of Cardiology*, September 2012, http://www.escardio.org/about/what/advocacy/EuroHeart/Pages/2012.

[113] Ibid.

stated that "The mantra that saturated fat must be removed to reduce the risk of cardiovascular disease has dominated dietary advice and guidelines for almost four decades. Yet scientific evidence shows that this advice has, paradoxically, increased our cardiovascular risks ..."[114]

So-called experts assure us that the "lipid hypothesis" is based on solid scientific research and indisputable evidence. Meanwhile, it turns out that such evidence is scarce, and its quality is often questionable.

The Framingham Heart Study (FHS) is the most well-known and respected clinical research in contemporary medicine. The results of the study have revealed high blood pressure to be one of the main risk factors for stroke, coronary heart disease, and heart and kidney failure. It is often cited in numerous publications as evidence confirming the "lipid hypothesis."

The study, the first phase of which began in 1948, included 5,209 participants of both sexes between the ages of thirty and sixty-two. In the second phase in 1971, the children of the initial participants along with their spouses were added in another group (5,124 persons). The third phase began in 2002, in which the grandchildren of the first group's participants took part.

According to this multiyear, thoroughly conducted project, then-director of the FHS Dr. William Castelli announced that "animal fat is not associated with heart disease." The

---

[114]   Dr. Mercola, "Heart Specialist Calls for Major Repositioning on Saturated Fat, as It's NOT the Cause of Heart Disease," Mercola.com, accessed November 4, 2013, http://articles.mercola.com/sites/articles/archive/2013/11/04/saturated-fat-intake.aspx.

research indicated that "the more saturated fat one ate, the more cholesterol one ate, the more calories one ate, the lower the person's serum cholesterol ... We found that the people who ate the most cholesterol, the most saturated fat, and the most calories weighed the least and were the most physically active."[115]

Toni Jeffreys's publication *Your Health at Risk* (1998) cites another researcher and former FHS director, Dr. William Kannel, who states that there was "no discernible association between the amount of cholesterol in the diet and the level of cholesterol in the blood regardless of how much or how little animal fat in the diet." The cholesterol you consume does not influence the amount of cholesterol in your blood.

The thorough and costly ($150 million) Lipid Research Clinics Coronary Primary Prevention Trial (LRC-CPPT) is often cited by experts justifying the need to introduce a low-fat diet. The patients participating in the study received low-fat, low-cholesterol food. The effect of saturated fats on their bodies was not studied, and neither were the effects of high levels of cholesterol, which their food did not contain.

The aim of this study was something completely different: to test the effectiveness of cholesterol-lowering medications! The data indicated a 24 percent reduction in CHD (coronary heart disease) in the group that took the medication. A decrease in the heart disease death rate was also observed. However, popular magazines and journals still reported the results of the LRC-CPPT study as showing that animal fat is the greatest killer in the world!

---

[115] William P. Castelli, "Concerning the Possibility of a Nut ..." *Archives of Internal Medicine* 152(7) (1992): 1371–2.

Human breast milk contains more cholesterol than any other food; 50 percent of its total fatty acids are saturated fat, which is essential for a child's proper development, particularly that of his or her brain (compare this with the diet of pregnant and breastfeeding Chinese women, discussed previously in the section on eggs). The common recommendations by "experts" of low-fat products for small children may thus come as a surprise.

The globally renowned Nurses' Health Studies began in 1976 and are now in their third generation, with a total of more than 275,000 participants. Former Secretary of the US Department of Health and Human Services Donna Shalala called NHS "one of the most significant studies ever conducted on the health of women." The studies were unusually long-term, trustworthy, and broad in scope, and their results have been published in over 265 scientific publications. The studies did not find a significant link between the consumption of saturated fats and cholesterol and heart disease. Many attempts have been made to undermine the studies' results, but not one has succeeded in proving that a high-fat diet (in itself) causes heart disease.

A meta-analysis from 2010 that collected data from twenty-one studies and included nearly 348,000 adults found no difference in the risks of coronary heart disease, stroke, and cardiovascular disease between people with the lowest and highest intakes of saturated fat.[116] Another 2010 study published in the *American Journal of Clinical Nutrition* found that replacing saturated fat with a higher carbohydrate

---

[116] *American Journal of Clinical Nutrition* 91(3) (March 2010): 535–46.

intake, particularly refined carbohydrates, exacerbates insulin resistance and obesity, increases triglycerides and small LDL particles, and reduces beneficial HDL cholesterol. According to the authors, any attempts to decrease your risk of cardiovascular disease through diet must recognize the *limitations of refined carbohydrate intake and weight reduction.*

The world stands in awe of Japanese longevity. The popular view is that their secret lies in their low-fat diet. This opinion falls apart when we take a closer look at the nation's eating habits.

The Japanese regularly consume eggs, pork, beef, poultry, seafood, and animal organs, as well as fruits and vegetables. Their favorite crustaceans and fish soup traditionally appear on their tables daily. They consume more cholesterol than most of us! Yet, they do not eat large amounts of vegetable oils, flour-based products, sugars, or processed foods.

They mainly use fresh, raw foods in their cuisine. They do not have a custom of preserving, freezing, or storing foods; instead, they consider food shopping to be a daily necessity! The Japanese are also famous for their calm, drawn-out meals, which are to be a feast not only for the body but also the soul. Their dishes are thus real works of art, and their colors, shape, and composition must be a source of beauty.

The Japanese themselves joke about this: "Is there any difference between a Chinese person and a Japanese person? Yes, plenty! The most important difference is that, when the Chinese person sees something moving or growing in nature, he or she thinks about how to eat it, while the Japanese person ponders how to eat it beautifully."

The Swiss are known in Europe and around the world for their longevity and excellent health and do not exclude fresh butter, eggs, various meats, and cream (as seen in the famed Swiss creamed espresso) from their diet. They've been on a high-fat diet for centuries! Meanwhile, in Italy and France, many decide what to have for dinner based on tradition and pleasure, eating so-called "unhealthy foods." Traveling in the South of France, you can (fortunately) see that the locals are not in such dire health straits as most Americans. We're probably all aware of the "French paradox," according to which people consuming foie gras and triple crème cheeses while drinking wine still stay slim and attractive.

Okinawa is home to many Japanese whose advanced age (over eighty years old) and good physical condition are nothing unusual. They are strong, fit, independent, and active, though some are already over a hundred. Heart disease, strokes, and cancer are rare. It is often stressed that the residents of Okinawa follow a primarily vegetarian, soy-based diet (e.g., miso paste, tofu, soy sauce). It is forgotten, however, that soy and other legumes make up only 6 percent of their diet. Just like in other regions of Japan, residents of Okinawa eat pork, and every part of the pig and its internal organs are considered culinary delicacies. Meat is generally eaten on weekends and holidays, while their everyday diet is based on fish, crustaceans, shellfish, and plants. Most dishes are made with lard. The island's residents exercise moderation in their eating habits; they don't overeat, and they eat nonimported fruit, vegetables, and seaweed. They consume lots of rice, fiber, and fish stock and, like other Japanese people, eat nearly no sugars, flour-based products, or processed, preserved, or frozen foods. Hydrogenated vegetable oils do not exist in their diet! They are very physically active: they tend to their gardens themselves, go on long hikes, and take care of their well-loved animals.

I imagine the material presented here has significantly undermined your previous ideas of a healthy diet. This information allows you to see that a healthy diet should provide the body with everything it needs to build, restore, and energize itself and should limit the appearance of toxic metabolic products and allow them to be removed efficiently. Saturated animal fats are necessary for these processes, as they are the greatest source of energy, but they are also burned.

This book is intended for readers who know how to decide for themselves and who want to acquire the information and skills that will allow them to improve their quality of life in a pleasant, fun, and knowledgeable way. If you've made it this far, you're certainly motivated to achieve this goal. If you find yourself doubting the information presented here, look at the original source materials, which present a broader view of the topics discussed here.

Fortunately, over the past decade, more research has been done criticizing the "lipid hypothesis." You can see this clearly by simply Googling "cholesterol skeptics"; you will find the International Network of Cholesterol Skeptics (or the Weston A. Price Foundation), which brings together eminent physicians and scientists from around the world working with unwavering courage to debunk the myth of cholesterol's lethal effects by using the latest research results.

Their experiments demonstrate beyond a doubt that atherosclerosis is caused primarily by the excessive oxidation of a certain type of cholesterol, which makes up only a small part of the valuable substances flowing through our bloodstream. Animal fats are nourishing, long-lasting, tasty, fragrant, and, most important, remarkably nutritious.

As biochemist Michael Gurr sums up in one of his articles, "Whatever causes coronary heart disease, it is not primarily a high intake of saturated fat."[117] It is easy to see that no authority, research, evidence, facts, or arguments have stopped the high priests of the "lipid hypothesis," who continue to lambast the greatest works of culinary art: butter, cream, omelets, soufflés, full-fat cheeses, juicy steaks, and pork hocks. Well, in politics and religion, ideas are mightier than an entire army!

Also you should know that high temperatures and oxygen can damage cholesterol (fats). In turn, damaged and oxidized cholesterol can wreak havoc on your artery walls. Foods containing damaged cholesterol should thus be avoided like the plague! Powdered eggs and milk, coffee creamers, mayonnaise, and candy made with powdered eggs, skim milk, and even yogurt are full of this bad cholesterol!

Everything has been turned upside down; people trying to escape from "lethal" cholesterol eat it in its most dangerous form, which is responsible for heart disease and many other conditions.

How dependent people must be on such myths and stereotypes! Their acceptance occurred so imperceptibly that it is hard for us to believe we've become victims of indoctrination and deceitful tricks. Most of us (unfortunately!) go through

---

[117] M. Gurr, "A Fresh Look at Dietary Recommendations," *Inform* 7(4) (June 1996): 432–435.

life convinced that we are more immune than others to such external influences and manipulation by our surroundings, advertisements, and the media.

Remember

- Organic, healthy fats are an excellent, efficient energy source and form the irreplaceable building blocks of the cells in our body.
- Hydrogenated fats should be eliminated from our diet, as they are detrimental to human health and can even be life-threatening.
- Animal fats play an important role in building and maintaining our reproductive readiness. In this way, they support a proper sex drive. A diminished or suppressed sex drive caused by diet can lead to unexpected and frustrating disruptions in this important area of human life.
- The cholesterol you consume does not influence the amount of cholesterol in your blood.
- A low-fat diet does not guarantee good health or longevity.
- The so-called lipid hypothesis is based on scarce evidence that has been questioned by the scientific community.
- People with low cholesterol suffer from coronary heart disease to the same degree as those with high cholesterol.

Why Omega 3?

Until relatively recently, talking about essential omega-3 and omega-6 fatty acids at a social function would have been unthinkable. It would have looked more like a chemistry conference than a conversation among people interested in a healthy diet.

Interest in these fatty acids began to grow in the 1970s, when studies were carried out on the Inuit diet. Two Danish scientists, Jorn Dyerberg and Hans Olaf Bang, noted this society suffered only rare instances of diabetes, psoriasis, atherosclerosis, heart attacks, and other cardiovascular diseases.[118] Their diet was based on oily cold-water fish.

It became an extremely hot topic at the time, yet nobody needs convincing of the benefits of such a diet today. Fish and seafood have been shown to be invaluable sources of high-quality protein, vitamins A and D, B vitamins, iron, calcium, phosphorus, copper, magnesium, potassium, sodium, and especially omega-3 and omega-6 fatty acids.

These days, dieticians around the world consider them to be one of the healthiest and best foods for the human body. A lack of such fish in our diet can lead to many diseases, while consuming them in appropriate amounts not only provides us with nutrients and energy, but also helps prevent and even treat such diseases, thanks to their omega-3 content.

The societies of the Mediterranean, Japan, and Greenland know this well. They've long seen how their wounds heal

---

[118] J. Dyerberg and H. O. Bang, "Haemostatic Function and Platelet Polyunsaturated Fatty Acids in Eskimos," *Lancet* 2(8140) (September 1979): 433–5, http://www. ncbi.nlm.nih.gov/pubmed/89498/.

faster, their kidneys and liver function better, and how they enjoy greater resistance to infections.

Today, we know that the average person's omega-3 requirement is about 1 to 1.5 grams daily and that we should eat saltwater fish at least twice a week. In addition, we should consume shrimp, crab, squid, and other *frutti di mare* more often, which many nations have known for centuries. There is one other benefit of such foods that has been known for thousands of years. Seafood has an excellent effect on the quality of our sex lives, as it is a highly effective aphrodisiac when eaten raw.

While we are generally aware of the role that vitamins and microelements play in the development and functioning of our body, we know relatively little about essential fatty acids (EFAs). Omega-3 is an exceptionally healthy and crucial fatty acid, and an omega-3 deficiency can contribute to or even cause serious health problems, both psychological and physical. It is estimated that such a deficiency is an underlying factor contributing to 96,000 premature deaths each year.[119] As an essential unsaturated fatty acid, omega-3 is not produced by the human body and must be provided by food. Many people do this by adding omega-3 supplements to their daily diet. This is one of the simplest and most effective ways we can improve our health.

I personally recommend krill oil supplements. Krill are a small crustacean found in colder waters, mainly off Antarctica.

[119] Dr. Mercola, "How Turning the Food Pyramid on Its Head Can Help You 'Slim Down without Trying,'" Mercola.com, June 22, 2013, http://articles.mercola.com/sites/articles/archive/2013/06/22/food-pyramid-guide.aspx.

They serve as a basic food source for whales and have also long been consumed by humans.

Krill are used by food producers in many countries, especially Japan and Russia. Their fats are rich in EFAs and water-soluble vitamins, particularly niacin, vitamin B_{12}, calcium, sulfur, magnesium, phosphorus, and iodine. Consuming the right amount of omega-3 has a beneficial effect on our cardiovascular system, ensures that our brain and immune system are functioning properly, and gives us healthy skin.

Studies show that omega-3 fatty acid consumption significantly lowers the level of triglycerides in the blood, reducing the risk of first-time and recurring heart attacks. It also significantly slows our cells' aging process. Some data emphasize the cancer-fighting properties of omega-3s and their beneficial impact on humans' psychological and intellectual development, as well as cognitive functioning. There are also studies that suggest omega-3 reduces the symptoms of depression and aggressive behavior. However, too much omega-3 can also be harmful. Therefore, it should be consumed in moderate amounts. Individuals who take anticoagulant drugs or have blood coagulation problems should avoid omega-3 supplementations, because omega 3 can affect blood clotting. According to Andrew Weil, MD, "Very high intakes of fish oil/omega-3 fatty acids may increase the risk of hemorrhagic stroke and have been associated with nosebleed and blood in the urine."[120]

---

[120] Weil, "Too Much Omega-3?" accessed April 20, 2018, https://www.drweil.com/vitamins-supplements-herbs/vitamins/too-much-omega-3/

We should also exercise considerable caution in this area because the production of items with omega-3 fatty acids has become a multibillion-dollar business: Americans spend $2.6 billion on average on dietary supplements containing omega-3.[121]

In my introduction, I mentioned some natural sources of omega-3 fats. Fish oil is one item on the market, but it is not the only source. This theory was spread by a very effective marketing campaign by the fishing industry lobby, which invested large amounts of money in taking over the market following the attack on red meat in the 1990s.

Red meat was blamed for causing heart disease, high blood pressure, high cholesterol, intestinal cancer, and so on. Taking advantage of the aggressive criticism of the meat industry, fish producers presented their products as a healthier alternative. Yet, the reality looks somewhat different. We have many possible ways of obtaining omega-3 fatty acids, which I will explain in the following section.

The Benefits of Omega 6

Omega-6 acids, like omega-3s, are essential unsaturated fatty acids and must also be obtained through food. The right ratio of omega-3 to omega-6 is vital to our health. Eating large amounts of omega-6 with a simultaneous deficiency in omega-3 contributes to the development of breast cancer in postmenopausal women.

---

[121] Dr. Mercola, "Are You Getting the Right Type of Omega-3 Fats?" Mercola.com, April 3, 2010, http://articles.mercola.com/sites/articles/archive/2010/04/03/are-you-getting-the-right-type-of-omega3-fats.aspx.

Arachidonic acids (AA, ARA), a type of omega-6 fatty acid, facilitate the production of proinflammatory hormones: prostaglandins. Meanwhile, omega-3 acids are anti-inflammatory in nature and compete with omega-6 acids in the body, lowering their concentration in our tissues and limiting their reactions with enzymes.

Omega-6 acids are present in nearly all the food products we buy: vegetable oils, animal fats, candies, baked goods, and many other snacks. Processed, hydrogenated fats also include omega-6 and are present in nearly all industrially produced food products. This has led to a seriously distorted ratio of omega-6 to omega-3. Mother Nature planned this ratio of omega-6 to omega-3 perfectly: 1 to 1, sometimes 2 to 1, and even 4 to 1. Meanwhile, in today's typical diet, this ratio rises to 20 to 1![122]

This ratio of omega-6 to omega-3 triggers a genetically programmed inflammatory response, which is part of our first line of biological defense against pain, infection, and injuries. Our body identifies and destroys toxic material in the damaged tissues and keeps it from spreading to our entire organism. Unfortunately, this ideally functioning system has become destabilized and has gotten out of control. This is due to poor eating habits, the arrogance of food producers, and the couldn't-care-less attitude of many food consumers.

If we add stress and a lack of physical activity to the mix, our disoriented body reacts as if it were under attack by a destructive enemy infection or had suffered a serious injury. And thus the disease process begins.

---

[122] Sisson, *The Primal Blueprint*, 83.

What Type of Omega-3 Should Be in Our Diet?

Most of the undeniable health benefits of omega-3 unsaturated fatty acids are related to the animal- and fish-based omega-3 fatty acid DHA (docosahexaenoic acid). DHA is valued for lowering blood triglyceride levels and protecting the heart. A diet deficient in DHA contributes to low levels of serotonin in the brain and may also be linked to the appearance of ADHD, Alzheimer's disease, and depression. A UCLA study published in the *American Journal of Geriatric Psychiatry* found that the Mediterranean diet (a diet rich in omega-3 fatty acids)[123] may help prevent the brain from developing the toxic plaques and tangles associated with Alzheimer's disease.

The omega-3 fatty acid ALA (alpha-linolenic acid) is found mainly in nuts and flaxseed and is used to enrich many of the food products offered in supermarkets, pharmacies, and health-food stores.

Cardiologists are convinced, however, that ALAs do not offer any health benefits, since our body only weakly converts ALA to EPA and DHA, and when it does, it is only on a very small scale. So, even if you eat large amounts of ALA omega-3s (flaxseed, hemp seeds, chia seeds, and walnuts), you should still supplement them with animal forms of omega-3s (raw, organic eggs; red meat from free-range animals; wild fish, krill, or cod liver oil; and farm-fresh butter).

The Japanese, for example, not only obtain omega-3s from animal sources but also by eating seaweeds, such as *wakame*,

---

[123] The Mediterranean diet boasts a rich variety of flavors and includes animal fats, dairy, meat, and eggs. Fatty fish is eaten on a regular basis. It also offers an assortment of traditionally fermented foods and some vegetables, which are often cooked with cream, olive oil, or lard.

kombu, and *nori*, which contain these fatty acids as well. They are also found in small amounts in leafy green vegetables, fresh herbs, and to a greater degree in pumpkin seeds.

We should also eat plenty of whole foods rich in vitamin E (my favorites are almonds, spinach, sweet potatoes, avocado, and butternut squash). Vitamin E helps us absorb omega-3, and this vitamin also fights the effects of oxidation.

Animal Sources of Omega-3 Fatty Acids

The health-conscious among us take special omega-3 supplements and give them to their loved ones daily. They rejoice that what was once the bane of their childhood existence—a forced-down spoonful of cod liver oil—is today a pleasure. But the colorful, flavored cod liver oil is not an acceptable way to take omega-3s. I would warn that these substances are full of chemical dyes and artificial flavors and fragrances. As such, they absolutely cannot be considered healthy! I recommend other methods of supplementation. Animal-source omega-3s can be found in many foods, and we should take care to keep them on our tables. The basic ones include fish (my favorites are sardines and anchovies), fish oils, cod liver oil, krill oil, organic free-range eggs, and red meat as well as fresh, organic butter.

1. **Fish.** Fish are certainly an excellent source of all types of omega-3, but (as I've written earlier) in their case, one should proceed with caution. Unfortunately, most of the fish we find are contaminated with industrial toxins, chemical waste, heavy metals, and radioactive

substances. It's a shame that a fish-based diet cannot be recommended these days as a long-term solution. Indeed, it's a great pity. But you can still add wild salmon, herring, mackerel, sardines, and anchovies to your diet, provided you pay close attention to their freshness and quality and make sure they are young, small fish. This is because such specimens have spent much less time in polluted water and are thus less full of toxins than older, larger fish.

2. **Fish Oils.** Fish oil is an excellent source of omega-3 fatty acids. It also has many other benefits. But it should be admitted that they are poor in antioxidants. This poses a certain problem because when we eat omega-3 fatty acids, we also need to be sure to provide antioxidant protection. This is necessary because fish oils spoil and oxidize incredibly easily (like all fish and seafood products), leading to the formation of harmful free radicals.

Fish oils should be consumed in combination with appropriate antioxidants, to prevent these destructive internal processes from taking place. We can then be certain that both are contributing to our good health. We should also remember that fish oil is only as good as the fish it comes from, and these days, well, suffice it to say, a good fish is hard to find.

3. **Cod Liver Oil.** Until recently, cod was one of the cheapest fish available (along with herring) and wasn't

considered a real delicacy. For that reason, cod were rarely sold fresh; they were more often smoked instead, so they could be offered for sale longer. Today, our attitude toward cod has changed completely.

International law regulates cod fishing by imposing defined limits and seasons on fishermen. They are harvested mainly as food, but the pharmaceutical industry has also played a major role. The production of cod liver oil in liquid and capsule form has made cod a marketable and even expensive fish because of its omega-3 content. Cod liver oil has a beneficial effect on our immune system and is a rich source of vitamins A and D. It is a much better source of omega-3 fatty acids than other fish oils.

4. **Krill Oil.** This really is the number-one source of omega-3 fatty acids! It contains forty-eight times more active antioxidants than any other fish oil. It also contains a unique flavonoid—astaxanthin— which binds EPA and DHA, thus enabling the most beneficial, direct metabolism of these antioxidants by making them more readily absorbed by our body.

These days, war could easily break out in the Antarctic over krill, if not for the fact that krill fishing is one of the best regulated procedures in the world. Strict international regulations, catch limits, and fishing seasons all ensure its stable growth. All decisions in this matter are subject to continuous review and verification. One can be sure that all krill products are fresh, since they are made directly onboard special processing ships at sea.

Their edible parts are cooked, crushed, pressed, and frozen into blocks, which are then transported to the appropriate specialist factories. Although this crustacean's taste makes it something of a minishrimp, it has taken several long, difficult years for it to appear on many nations' tables. And how things have changed! Anyone who can fight for krill will!

5. **Red Meat and More.** Studies have shown that organic, free-range, grass-fed meat has a high omega-3 fatty acid content. This is also true of milk products from such animals.

6. **Butter.** Butter should have a lovely, deep-yellow color, which indicates that it is produced from the milk of healthy cows. Only this type of butter boasts high amounts of omega-3 and omega-6 fatty acids in ideal proportions to one another. It is also rich in vitamins A and D.

7. **Eggs.** Their yolks provide large amounts of choline and omega-3 and omega-6 fatty acids in the right proportions. Again, I recommend *kogel mogel* as an incredibly nutritious dessert that can be made by anyone, anywhere (I have described it in an earlier chapter).

I hope this list of foods will help you find your way through the world of advertising, which doesn't always give us reliable information on the quality and value of our food. The omega-3 and omega-6 fatty acids discussed here and the foods that contain them are undoubtedly crucial to our health, and introducing them into our diet is an obvious choice.

The rules of healthy eating are actually quite clear and simple. Our health is a direct reflection of our lifestyle, and diet is its most important factor. Our diet should thus consist of nutritious, organic food, raised and produced in a natural and responsible way, without genetic modifications or toxic chemicals.

There's no way that genetically modified crops raised using tons of chemical substances or factory-farmed animals pumped full of hormones and antibiotics could provide healthy raw materials for producing food, which, in turn, is further processed, pasteurized, irradiated, dyed, hardened, ground up, and filled with "enhancers," fragrances, and added preservatives. It's not possible for this system to produce something good or beneficial for us to eat.

We can't eat such junk and then fill in the gaps with synthetic vitamins and artificial supplements of everything these unsafe foods lack. That's not the right way to achieve truly radiant health. Providing individual nutrients to our body separately completely misses the mark!

Separating out vitamins, then minerals, then protein, then ... what is this mess? For our bodies to function optimally, we need many different types of food to provide the raw materials for the numerous biochemical processes taking place in our system. Aggressive supplementation can become yet another problem on top of any nutritional deficiencies and may cause a serious disruption in the way the body works.

Learning a few rules and accepting some kind, tried-and-true advice can make a happy, fully satisfying life yours. Nature can't be fooled, and any such irresponsible attempts will certainly come back to haunt us.

* * *

I've been visiting Russia quite often for a while now, and there, I've had the pleasure of tasting the exceptional regional delicacy known as *salo*. It is a special type of cured, coarse-salted pork fat, which is cooked over a low flame for about 30 minutes, with many different seasonings rubbed in beforehand.

After cooling, salo is cut into thin strips and eaten with any type of bread (though Russian-style black bread is best) or is enjoyed on its own to better savor its unique delicacy and exceptional taste. Salo is sometimes served with pickles, onions, or garlic, which are served with vodka as "necessary liver support." This pork fat—several inches thick—is obtained from healthy, organically raised pigs.

It is alabaster white and has a firm, dense consistency. Salo has become popular not only in Ukraine but also Russia and Belarus, and those repatriated after World War II from the eastern borderlands of the prewar Second Polish Republic to the western areas of today's Poland have kept the secrets of its production to this day.

Folks use it like bacon in many regional dishes: borscht, potato pancakes, sauerkraut soup, scrambled eggs, and bean and pea soups. Considering that pork fat is one of the richest sources of vitamin D available, adding salo to our diet can help us get through those long, cold winter evenings. I assure you that it is wonderfully aromatic, healthy, and tasty, and it's worth having on your table. It's absolute poetry!

Remember

- Damaged and oxidized cholesterol can wreak havoc on your artery walls. Powdered eggs and milk, coffee creamers, mayonnaise, and candy made with powdered eggs, skim milk, and even yogurt are full of this bad cholesterol!
- Omega-3 and omega-6 fatty acids are natural sources of health and longevity, protecting us against heart disease, atherosclerosis, depression, dementia, and so on.
- These fatty acids have a beneficial effect when they are found in the right proportions of omega-6 to omega-3: one-to-one, two-to-one, and four-to-one ratios.
- To make sure you're getting enough healthy fats, try to eat avocados, raw dairy products, raw nuts, and olive oil and also add a high-quality source of animal-based omega-3s, such as krill oil.

CHAPTER 9

A CHEAT SHEET

Every day, we eat a certain portion of food without realizing that over the course of an entire year, this amount builds up to around one ton of food, which must provide energy, building materials, and vitality to the seventy trillion cells that make up the structure of the average human being! Our food allows innumerable biochemical processes to take place in our body, which we can thank for keeping us alive. In a world in which the cynical pursuit of profit has taken over food production and led to industrial-scale agriculture and factory farms, we should become aware of what that ton of food contains and what is delivered to each of our trillions of cells!

Many of the thoughts of French Enlightenment lawyer, writer, and gastronome Jean Anthelme Brillat-Savarin in his famous work *The Physiology of Taste* (admired by Honoré de Balzac, among others) remain relevant warnings and tips for today's food consumers. Some of them have become timeless, stand-alone aphorisms, and those who quote them may not always know that they came from this master of French culinary literature: "Tell me what you eat, and I will tell you what you are" and "The fate of a nation depends on the way that its people eat."

By checking to ensure the quality of our food and its ingredients and origin, we demonstrate responsibility for our health and lives! By refusing to eat preserved, industrially processed, chemically "enhanced," and generally suspicious foods, we support the brave yet essential aspiration of conscious consumers to eliminate low-quality food from our supermarket shelves.

But how does this look in day-to-day life? Is it possible to formulate fixed, concrete, and detailed rules in this respect? Can we find proper, organic food uncontaminated by chemicals without having this search become a burdensome obligation that sucks all the joy out of eating? What should guide us, when there are so many mutually exclusive ideas about how to treat and prevent many diseases (including the diseases of civilization) that recommend fat-free cooking (boiling or steaming), as well as a traditional high-fat diet? How can you find your bearings in this chaos of information without being a specialist? You've got to bring your common sense, a bag, and a cheat sheet on your shopping trips!

A cheat sheet (that learning aid known to students in every school around the world) is essential for finding healthy food. It will serve as a warning to keep us from buying the toxic products that pose an ever-growing danger to us. It highlights many concerning facts that we hadn't thought about before, instead treating them as normal and obvious.

Regardless of the time, place, or level of civilization, acquiring food has been, is, and will continue to be a fundamental problem for humans, tied to the fear of not only hunger and weakness but, above all, losing one's health and life. In addition to these aspects, I, a self-proclaimed sybarite and epicure, am also convinced by the delight and pleasure that fresh, fragrant, and organic food provides to my palate.

For my loved ones, close friends, and me, enjoying meals and meeting and conversing at the table have a unique power and significance. It's not just the clinking of the silverware, the wafting aromas, and the exquisite flavors. It's also about maintaining interpersonal ties, good humor, anecdotes, and aesthetic experience.

This attitude to food goes along with the thought of the connoisseur Brillat-Savarin mentioned earlier: "The pleasures of the table are for every human, of every land, and no matter of what place in history or society. They can be a part of all his (or her) other pleasures, and they last the longest, to console him (or her) when he (or she) has outlived the rest."

So, what should we pay attention to so that these pleasures, enhanced by real, nutritious food, can always be found on our tables? To help you, I provide mini cheat sheets which can serve you as a guide while shopping for nutritious food in the appendix section in this book.

CHAPTER 10

DAIRY: WHITE MADNESS

As late as the 1970s, fresh milk was still associated with the clinking of glass bottles at the door, the milkman ringing the doorbell, and, of course, having to get up early to meet him. Anyone who'd had a bit too much to drink the night before thankfully greeted the milk and milkman even at the crack of dawn!

I use the term *milk* here in general, as EU law currently dictates that the single word be used only for cow's milk. Milk from other animals must include an additional descriptive term: sheep's milk, goat's milk, and so on.

Milk has been an essential part of our diet for centuries, as it was widely considered to be exceptionally nutritious because of the presence of nearly all the necessary nutrients in it and in an easily assimilated form to boot. It is said that a single quart of milk meets our daily requirements of calcium and vitamins A, B1, and B2, as well as vitamin D, which is essential for strong bones.

It's openly acknowledged, however, that milk contains very little iron, vitamin C, and niacin. The presence of vitamins in milk depends on several factors but, above all, on the cows' diet and how much time they spend outside in sunny pastures (vitamin D).

Traditionally, milk is thought to be healthy for everyone, end of story! In the past, it seemed that thorough studies of milk were just a formality, and there was no doubt that such opinions would be confirmed. However, that didn't happen. The debate over milk has been sparked for good, and it continues to become more and more heated to this day! Truth be told, no other product has aroused such controversy and conflict within the scientific community. So, what is it all about, and what are milk's supporters and detractors really dealing with?

Milk is a substance secreted from the mammary gland of all female mammals during lactation. It's a complex mixture with many different components. Chemically speaking, it's an emulsion of fats with water, containing protein, vitamins, and mineral substances.

Its quality and nutritional value is 70 percent determined by environmental factors, such as the individual animal's living conditions and food, and 30 percent by the animal's physical predispositions. That's why each mammal's milk is different, and only some types can be directly consumed by humans.

For thousands of years, cow's milk has been the most important, though in many geographical regions, the milk of goats, buffalo, sheep, camels, reindeer, llamas, yaks, and even donkeys and mares is also consumed. Each is considered to have exceptional nutritional and even medical value. What's more, each has been present in the food culture of its respective society since time immemorial.

History has given us abundant evidence of the high regard in which milk was once held as a food source. The early Slavs included it in their offerings to the gods and protective household deities, thanking them for a plentiful harvest and peaceful existence. They poured small amounts of it into tiny bowls, which they would set on the threshold of their homes. The ancient Greeks worshipped milk as a gift from the gods and saw "white, spilled patches" of it in the heavens. They called the stars and nebulas they saw *galaktikos*, or milky.

But milk was not part of a daily diet everywhere, much less used in ritual worship. In some cultures, milk is completely absent from the human diet, as it can't be digested. These include Chinese and Japanese societies, the societies of the Polynesian islands, and the Aboriginal cultures, and it is only rarely consumed by Arabs in the Middle East.

Today, there is perhaps no continent on Earth where the dairy industry hasn't begun to produce, purchase, store, process, and distribute milk on a large scale. The foundations of this were set by our nomadic hunter-gatherer ancestors, who spread this "white blood" and valued it for its great life- and health-giving properties.

However, as I recall those times when nobody had any doubts as to milk's healthy nature, I should also present opinions that are a far cry from these positive evaluations. It is hard to believe that only a few decades ago, people accepted such positive views without question.

Today, just like fat, milk is held responsible for nearly every health problem, from ear infections to cancer to diabetes. Along with sugar, salt, and white bread, it is one of the "bad white foods" threatening humanity.

Publications have come out with titles meant to scare the public. The Indian physician and proponent of vegetarianism Nand Kishore Sharma is the author of the book *Milk: A Silent Killer*, in which, as the title suggests, he claims it is extremely harmful to humans, accusing milk of causing heart disease.

In his book *Please, Don't Drink Your Milk*, American physician Frank A. Oski states that any person who is able to process solid food should never consume milk, especially not pasteurized milk. The ear, nose, and throat specialist Dr. Fred Pullen, along with Dr. Michael Schmidt, is sure that it's responsible for recurring ear infections, intestinal distress, acne, and intense menstrual pain among girls and women.

So, what is the truth about milk, whose production and consumption continues to rise? Does it really harm people's health and threaten our lives? Why is milk, with its sweet taste, a source of such deep dietary prejudices among so many people? Why do the Finns have such a long life expectancy, when they are first in the world in terms of milk and dairy consumption (with the Swedes, Dutch, and Swiss ranking next on the list)?

White Eminence with a (Recently!) Dark Reputation

Some people have a sensitivity to milk, which can appear in various ways (e.g., severe diarrhea) and thus lead to many different illnesses. This is most often caused by a deficiency in the enzyme lactase, which aids in the digestion of lactose, or milk sugar.[124] All infant mammals produce this enzyme, but, for most of them, this process disappears after they stop breastfeeding around two to four years of age.

Humans are the only mammals who drink milk by choice in adulthood and from a different creature to boot. Every female mammal produces milk with the right ingredients and in the correct proportions for the growth of her offspring, which differ from those of human breast milk and the needs of human children. Yet, 30 to 40 percent of societies on earth have retained the recessive gene that allows their bodies to continue to produce lactase into adulthood.[125]

These people come primarily from cultures that have consumed milk for millennia. The process of natural selection has decided who gets this necessary enzyme and who doesn't. Milk intolerance can also be caused by overuse of antibiotics.[126]

Many people are unaware that what they are allergic to is milk protein (casein), which is one of the most difficult-to-digest proteins in our body. It has properties that can trigger an autoimmune response and may cause allergic reactions that lead to serious health problems.

Following Keith Woodford's *Devil in the Milk* (2007), concern has grown over the A1 and A2 beta-casein content in milk (A1 and A2 cows). A2 beta-casein is the safe, nutritious protein form cows have produced since before they were first domesticated over ten thousand years ago. Yet a genetic

---

[124] Cow's milk is about 85 percent water. The remaining 15 percent is the milk sugar lactose, protein, fat, and minerals. The protein portion is 80 percent casein and 20 percent whey.

[125] Fallon and Enig, *Nourishing Traditions*, 33.

[126] "Mother's and offspring's use of antibiotics and infant allergy to cow's milk," accessed April 20, 2017, https://www.ncbi.nlm.nih.gov/pubmed/23348066.

mutation occurred in some European dairy herds that changed the beta-casein they produced. This change, which forms A1 beta-casein, allows a digestive enzyme to cut out a 7-amino-acid segment of the protein, a phenomenon that does not occur or occurs at a low rate with the older, safer A2 beta-casein. The 7-amino-acid segment that is separated from A1 beta-casein is known as *beta-casomorphin-7*, or BCM-7. It is an exogenous opioid (i.e., an opioid that doesn't naturally occur in the human body) that interacts with the human digestive system, internal organs, and brain stem. Its structure, similar to morphine, has been linked to autism and schizophrenia.[127] This protein may also create a shortage of antioxidants in the brain, also connected to autism.[128]

A1 beta-casein is common in many of the big black-and-white European cow breeds (e.g., Holstein and Friesian). Because of their size and milk production, these breeds produce the vast majority of milk available in Europe and America. However, I recommend cow's milk and milk products from older breeds like Jersey and Guernsey cows, which are genetically around 10 percent A1 and 90 percent A2.

Allowing milk to sour or ferment makes casein easier to digest. These processes change milk into a product with a wealth of beneficial bacteria, which make it possible to change milk sugar—lactose—into lactic acid.

[127] Josh Axe, *Eat Dirt: Eat Dirt: Why Leaky Gut May Be the Root Cause of Your Health Problems and 5 Surprising Steps to Cure It* (New York: HarperCollins, 2016), 73.
[128] Josh Harkinson, "You're Drinking the Wrong Kind of Milk," *Mother Jones*, March 12, 2014, http://www.motherjones.com/environment/2014/03/a1-milk-a2-milk-america. See also Axe, *Eat Dirt*, 73.

The final products of this fermentation, such as yogurt, kefir, farmer's cheese, and other cheeses are tolerated even by those adults who have had to cut milk out of their diet. It is also interesting that heavy cream and natural, traditional butter contain only small amounts of lactose and casein and are usually well tolerated and digested without any problems. For me, this is great news: butter and cream simply make everything taste better.

For those who have serious problems even with the products described here, I recommend the clarified butter product *ghee*, from which the milk solids have been completely removed. It is great for frying and unconditionally counts as a healthy fat.

When discussing popular dairy products that have been eaten through the ages, one can't forget about cheese. Cheeses that are not industrially processed and which are produced from unpasteurized milk have a complete set of enzymes and do not cause health problems even for those who have a low tolerance for dairy.

Aged cheeses are created via fermentation and thus contain very little lactose; they are well tolerated even by those sensitive to it. They are a real treasure trove of nutrients, as they contain high-quality fats and proteins, beneficial live bacterial cultures, vitamins, and minerals and are incredibly delicious besides. Processed cheeses bought at the supermarket (even the more expensive ones pretending to be delicacies) have no real nutritional value because of the high amounts of phosphates, hydrogenated oils, preservatives, and suspicious chemical cocktails that are found in them. They should be eliminated from our diet!

Even those who are genetically endowed with the ability to consume milk and dairy products without any problems *should never consume pasteurized milk* or products made from it. A study published in the *Journal of Agricultural and Food Chemistry* notes that a single glass of pasteurized milk can contain up to twenty different chemicals (besides growth hormones and antibiotics).[129]

Some people are convinced that pasteurization is necessary, since it protects consumers from dangerous illnesses. However, a closer analysis would indicate that the benefits of pasteurization have been grossly overstated.

Pasteurization was originally introduced as a temporary measure in 1800 CE[130] to create a sanitary barrier that would prevent the deaths of people living in urban regions. In those times, people raised cattle even in cities, in unimaginable filth and scandalous sanitary conditions, feeding the animals leftovers and slop from breweries. There were no standards for sterile milking or milk storage.

Milk at the time was not only highly contaminated but also watered down and grayish-blue (chalk was even added to obtain the desired white color!). The death rate for children at the time was over 50 percent.[131]

However, the facts presented here belong to the past, and the dairy industry has since developed such restrictive standards for each stage of contact with milk and dairy products that pasteurization for sanitary purposes is no longer necessary. Modern, mechanized systems for milking,

---

[129] Axe, *Eat Dirt*, 72.
[130] Ronald F. Schmid, *The Untold Story of Milk* (New Trends Publishing, 2003).
[131] Enig and Fallon, *Eat Fat Lose Fat*, 86.

stainless-steel containers, properly sealed packaging, and a well-controlled distribution system are enough to ensure the quality of our milk. What's more, these rules and the technology that comes with them had already been developed in 1940.

It should also be added that pasteurization (80°C–90°C) doesn't completely guarantee a sterile product, as shown by cases of salmonella poisoning caused by contaminated milk. In 1985, such incidences affected 14,000 residents of Illinois, while the strain of salmonella present in the pasteurized milk turned out to be genetically resistant to penicillin and tetracycline![132] Another ice cream-related outbreak occurred in the United States in 1994 and may have affected as many as 224,000 people.

Here's where the truth about raw milk gets lost, leaving consumers with misinformation rather than an accurate look at the data on milk safety. The CDC warns people not to consume raw milk because it may contain disease-causing bacteria.[133] However, this bacteria is not found in the raw milk produced by small, organic farmers. Rather, it is found in milk from the diseased animals that are the product of industrial farming practices. Take the industrial dairy farming methods out of the equation, and the bacteria never develops. The CEO of Organic Pastures Dairy, Mark McAfee, conducted an investigation that looked at the CDC's

---

[132] William Campbell Douglass, *The Milk Book: How Science Is Destroying Nature's Nearly Perfect Food* (Atlanta, GA: Second Opinion Publishing, 1994). See also Fallon and Enig, *Nourishing Traditions*, 34.

[133] https://www.cdc.gov/foodsafety/rawmilk/rawmilk-outbreaks.html.

own data on raw-milk-related deaths.[134] It turns out there are no deaths directly related to raw milk produced in the United States. The two deaths that the CDC lists as being related to raw milk occurred because people consumed illegal Mexican bathtub cheese, not US-produced raw milk. Also, more people become ill from drinking contaminated pasteurized milk than raw milk. A Cornell Study identified 1,100 cases of illness from raw milk compared to 422,000 from pasteurized milk from the same thirty-six-year period.

Pasteurization also fails to stop some other negative phenomena tied to milk. In the past, a normal, healthy cow produced from seven to eleven liters (around two to three gallons) of milk a day. Today, specially bred dairy cattle (Holstein and Friesian cattle) produce three to four times that amount. These creatures have abnormally active pituitary glands, which produce hormones that trigger the production of milk and EGF (epidermal growth factor), a factor that stimulates growth, including cellular growth and thus cancer cells as well.

In the 1970s, scientists determined which gene in cattle controls or codes for the production of bST. Bovine somatotropin (bST) is a growth hormone found in cattle. It thus became possible to synthesize the hormone and create recombinant bovine somatotropin (rBST) and recombinant bovine growth hormone (rBGH), or artificial growth hormone.

---

[134]   Mark McAfee Letter to CDC, accessed May 9, 2018, http://www.realmilk.com/commentary/mark-mcafee-letter-to-cdc/ via Mercola, "Raw Milk and Cheese Are Undergoing a Renaissance as Artisanal Foods Rise in Popularity," https://articles.mercola.com/sites/articles/archive/2016/04/16/raw-vs-organic-milk.aspx.

The FDA approved the use of the genetically engineered peptide hormones rBGH and rBST on dairy cows, and Monsanto was the first company to receive this approval. Mexico, Brazil, India, Russia, and at least ten other countries also approved rBST for commercial use.

Since 2000, rBST has been banned from the market in Canada, Australia, New Zealand, Japan, Israel, and the European Union. Argentina has also made it illegal to use rBST. But the FDA and the National Institutes of Health still assure consumers that dairy products and meat from cows treated with artificial growth hormone are safe for human consumption.

This doesn't bode well for us. While a small amount of this substance provided to calves in their mother's milk is necessary for the offspring to grow, in larger quantities, it becomes a source of numerous dysfunctions in both animals and people. As a European Union report on the animal welfare consequences of rBST states, its use often results in "severe and unnecessary pain, suffering and distress" for cows, which is connected with "serious mastitis, foot disorders and some reproductive problems."[135]

Scientists have also linked the substance's presence in milk to cancer.[136] Animals given this hormone are susceptible to various types of illnesses. As such, they are continually administered antibiotics and other pharmaceuticals that

---

[135] *Report on Animal Welfare Aspects of the Use of Bovine Somatotrophin*, the Scientific Committee on Animal Health and Animal Welfare, European Union, March 10, 1999, accessed January 16, 2008.

[136] Edward Group, "8 Shocking Facts about Bovine Growth Hormone," accessed May 14, 2016, https://www.globalhealingcenter.com/ natural-health/8-shocking-facts-bovine-growth-hormone/.

later become part of the milk we drink. Researchers at the University of Jaen in Spain also found traces of such drugs as niflumic acid, mefenamic acid, flunixin, diclofenac, ketoprofen, and ibuprofen, all of which are commonly used on the animals as painkillers.[137]

Let's avoid any negative outcomes by consuming milk and dairy products from healthy A2 cows pastured in meadows (especially during spring) and fed fresh, green herbs and grass, which contain numerous minerals and vitamins and cancer-fighting CLA.

The term *UHT* often appears on milk packaging. This is an abbreviation for "ultra-high temperature processing," which means sterilizing food products by quickly heating them to extremely high temperatures for one to two seconds and then immediately cooling them. This is also done with milk (132°C to 150°C).

The process destroys any bacteria while maintaining the food's original taste and smell. Unfortunately, at temperatures over 130°C, the product loses much of its nutritional value, which is then added back to the milk with artificial supplements. An analogous process is carried out using steam (at a temperature fluctuating between 130°C and 160°C) sent through a layer of milk over the course of one second, after which the milk is abruptly cooled.

Such milk, once opened, doesn't spoil for three months! It makes its way onto store shelves, and, since such milk has attracted the criticism of doctors and dieticians, the dairy industry has decided to change these opinions. How? By

---

[137]   Axe, *Eat Dirt*, 72.

using ever-changing technology meant to convince us that the final product is safe, fragrant, and delicious.

Cartons labeled "filtered milk" and "acidophilus milk" have now appeared on the market. The former is subjected to a long-term process of microfiltration, which involves straining the milk through thick, extremely fine filters (membranes), which are meant to catch bacteria and contaminants. The final white substance smells like milk and, like raw milk, remains fresh for only a short time (around forty-eight hours in the fridge) but is just as sterile as the other types mentioned.

The latest novelty, acidophilus milk, is nothing more than pasteurized milk to which producers have reintroduced the beneficial bacteria *Lactobacillus acidophilus*, which had previously been removed! The bacteria are meant to improve the product's nutritional value and help make any reintroduced vitamins easier to absorb.

This milk also has less lactose and must be consumed within four to five days. These methods are treated by dairy industry investors and businesspeople as a means of consoling those interested in the long-term safety of this basic raw material, which quickly spoils in nature. Whether they also have the good of consumers in mind, you can decide for yourself.

Raw, unpasteurized milk contains lactic acid bacteria, which protect against pathogens, as well as unusually beneficial enzymes, which, at the right pH (acidity), are activated in the intestines, aiding digestion and calcium absorption.

The pasteurization and UHT processes damage these highly beneficial organisms, and the final product is left completely defenseless, deprived of any sort of life—that is, sterile. In such a situation, our body must work much harder to process and break down the protein, sugar, and fat found in the milk. Digesting this milk places an unnecessary burden on the pancreas, forcing it to produce excessive amounts of enzymes, which can then lead to diabetes.

Heating milk to such high temperatures causes the undesirable modification of the amino acids lysine and tyrosine. The milk's protein becomes less available to the body as more weakly bioavailable, unsaturated fatty acids and vitamins are also damaged, and calcium, magnesium, phosphorus, potassium, and sulfur are almost eliminated.

In the face of such facts, the conviction that drinking pasteurized milk provides our body with the calcium needed for strong bones and teeth becomes plainly false! Healthy, injury- and disease-resistant bones also need phosphorus, magnesium, vitamin D, and vitamin K2, which almost completely disappear following pasteurization and UHT.

Pasteurized milk leads to weaker bones. This happens because the proportions of calcium to phosphorus are distorted: rather than 1 to 1, this ratio changes to 1 to 2.[138] To return to equilibrium, your body makes up for the lack of calcium by taking it from your bones. The result may be osteoporosis.

Calcium can be delivered to the body in two ways: either through ready-made supplements, or through a good diet. I obviously recommend the latter method and suggest introducing seeds, eggs, radishes, cocoa, buckwheat groats,

---

138   Richard De Leth, OERsterk (The Netherlands: Uitgeverij De Leth, 2012), 135.

cruciferous vegetables, asparagus, salmon, dried figs, tahini (sesame paste), fresh broths, and so on to your diet.

Another tried and true method for strengthening our bones is physical activity, which, depending on a variety of factors, can include walking, exercises, swimming, weightlifting, working in the garden, and many others (anything besides sitting on the couch in front of a computer or TV and washing down supplements with *fake milk*)!

The dairy industry continues to try to hoodwink consumers into buying the goods they offer. They add all sorts of chemicals to improve their quality, aroma, and color. They sprinkle in synthetic forms of vitamin D_2 or D_3, yet scientists and dieticians warn that synthetic vitamin D has the opposite effect of its natural counterpart. It causes softening of the bones and the hardening of soft tissues, such as your arteries.

Following such alarming observations, dairy industry experts removed vitamin D_2 and replaced it with D_3. Synthetic vitamin D_2, however, continues to be added to soy and rice milk.

All reduced-fat milk products are incredibly harmful to our health, particularly milk ranging from 0.5% to 2% milkfat. Such products are produced using powdered milk, which is made by boiling off the water to a level of only 2 to 3 percent of the final product, which is nothing more than oxidized cholesterol and can damage your arteries. The high temperatures used to dry milk (over hot metal rollers or by a stream of hot air) lead to the production of large amounts of burned protein and nitrates, which are dangerous carcinogens, as well as free glutamic acid, which is toxic to the nervous system.

Pasteurized, UHT, and reduced-fat milk is devoid of any sort of enzymes necessary for digestion and are therefore a burden on the digestive processes taking place in the human organism. Among people of advanced age, people with food intolerances, people with congenital digestive system disorders, infants, and older children, such milk makes its way through the system without being processed in the stomach.

It eventually settles around the tiny villi of the small intestine, coating and sealing them off, thereby making absorption of necessary minerals, vitamins, and microelements impossible. It also contributes to the secretion of toxic substances. This leads to allergies, chronic fatigue, and many other degenerative diseases.

There is yet another technological means of processing milk and dairy products that we should discuss: *homogenization*. This process results in a uniform mixture (hence the name, as the Greek word *homogenes* means "of the same kind") of individual components that do not naturally blend together into a single substance.

Milk, cream, and curd cheeses are homogenized to break up the fat globules in them so that they don't collect on the surface of the product. This process is carried out in high-pressure or rotary homogenizers, which reduce the fat molecules to at least a tenth of their original size and distribute them throughout the suspension. The technology makes the fat and cholesterol in the products highly susceptible to oxidation and rancidity. They thus become hazardous to our health.

Some scientific studies indicate that homogenized fat may be one of the causes of heart disease, as the broken-down molecules are not processed in the digestive system but enter directly into the bloodstream, thereby initiating many health problems.[139] Pasteurized, UHT, and homogenized milk and the dairy products made from them should never make it onto our tables, let alone into our stomachs!

I don't generally drink milk. If I do, I only drink the raw, organic, fermented kind, ideally made from goat's and sheep's milk. After all, milk and dairy cannot only be good sources of nutrition but also real pleasures. Some farms even supplement their raw milk with colostrum (the extra rich, "first run" milk that provides even more vitamins and nutrients), resulting in a lower-carb, higher-fat, higher-protein product. I adore kefir, yogurt, cream, butter, buttermilk, and whey. All these are made from raw milk and have existed in many cultures for a long time. Kefir, for example, is a fermented beverage originally from the Caucasus. It was apparently made in leather bags or oak barrels. The Armenians knew the secrets of its production even in ancient times, calling it *matsun* (English: matzoon). The drink is prized not only for its refreshing taste but also its beneficial impact on the digestive process.

Another product worthy of special attention is buttermilk, which is a dairy drink obtained while churning butter from cream. It increases the secretion of stomach juices, regulates digestion, and contains lactic acid. It is a wonderful way to quench your thirst on a hot day. It has a natural, slightly tart taste and pairs wonderfully (like kefir!) with fresh chopped or blended fruit.

---

[139] Mary Enig, "Milk Homogenization and Heart Disease," accessed September 20, 2016, https://www.westonaprice.org/health-topics/know-your-fats/milk-homogenization-heart-disease/.

I also recommend whey, which amateurs treat as a mere by-product of cheese and casein production. This translucent, slightly cloudy liquid is an excellent fortifying drink, which is especially tasty if you sprinkle in some coarse sea salt!

In ancient times, whey was valued as a highly effective detoxifying substance, as its cysteine content enables cells to produce glutathione, which performs a detoxifying function. It's perfect for a hangover. In the United States, whey is officially listed as a dermatologic agent, as it speeds up the healing process for burns and soothes burn-related pain. In such cases, it is applied externally in the form of whey-soaked compresses. In the heat of summer, it comes in handy in any form: as a drink and as a medication.

Cheese and the methods of its production have been known to humans for thousands of years, and it is one of the oldest food products made by humankind. Allusions to cheese can be found in the historical traditions of many ancient cultures, such as the ancient Greeks, Egyptians, Babylonians, Assyrians, and Romans.

Aristotle's writings included information on cheese production, and the Greek myths include the tale of its discovery by Aristaeus, king of Arcadia. Cheese was made in various, often quite primitive, conditions, as it served as food for Roman soldiers and was also consumed by Athenian athletes preparing for competitions and fights.

The secrets of the recipes and technology used were passed down from generation to generation over centuries. But the huge production lines of dairy businesses have managed to quickly obviate these efforts and have destroyed most of the small cheese houses and craft cheeseries around the world.

As health-conscious consumers, we should take care of those small cheese manufacturers that have been saved and work toward reopening those that have been closed. Only then will it be easier to find organic, raw milk and wonderful, healthy cheese.

Unpasteurized milk is extremely difficult to find in urban markets. It should be sought out among trusted farmers whose cattle are subjected to systematic veterinary checkups and are free of dangerous diseases like tuberculosis, brucellosis, or diphtheria and whose cowsheds are completely sanitary. Dr. Mercola stated that "drinking unpasteurized milk from cows raised in a CAFO (confined animal feeding operation) can be extremely dangerous and is not recommended under any circumstance."[140]

Unpasteurized milk should come from places where the animals are kept in humane conditions, allowed to graze in meadows, and fed healthy, fresh grass, while the milk should be obtained via mechanized milking equipment and stored in stainless steel containers at low temperatures. Such places do still exist and are worth finding!

***

While working on this chapter on dairy, I just so happened to receive a surprise gift from good friends returning from a trip to Ukraine: a fascinating, beautiful, four-volume work by Włodzimierz Szuchiewicz on a Ukrainian ethnic minority called the Hutsuls, titled *Huculszczyzna*, or *Hutsul Country*.

---

[140] Mercola, "Raw Milk and Cheese Are Undergoing a Renaissance as Artisanal Foods Rise in Popularity," accessed May 7, 2018, https://articles.mercola.com/sites/articles/archive/2016/04/16/raw-vs-organic-milk.aspx.

The book was published in 1902 and was commissioned by Count Włodzimierz Dzieduszycki, founder of the Dzieduszycki Museum of Natural History in Lviv.

In the first volume, I not only found descriptions of and recipes for Hutsul dishes using milk but also an intimate knowledge of this cottage industry. I was amazed by the extraordinarily simple Hutsul dishes, which, besides corn and lamb, are primarily based on milk and its products.

These Carpathian highlanders (around 300,000 people) living in southwestern Ukraine turned out to be quite creative in the kitchen. Their practices of raising sheep and cattle, herding, and growing small crops made their cuisine a truly fascinating phenomenon.

Besides frying scrambled eggs with sweet and sour cream, they made a nutritious, wonderfully warming soup from fresh milk with a bit of corn flour and added sour cream to boiled and cooled milk to make thick *huslanka*, a type of yogurt that could sit for half a year in a clay or wooden container. Whenever they felt like having a bit of this last delicacy, they just thinned some out with water or fresh milk. It was a nutritious food source not only for people, but also for cows and sheep after giving birth.

It is hard to believe that they could produce and store these dairy products in such primitive conditions, without preservatives, refrigerators, or complicated industrial processes!

Friends who have traveled there say that these wonderful people still make butter in so-called *faska*, or small wooden buckets, which they energetically shake, or by using long, wooden churns. In the latter, they beat the cream by rhythmically plunging poles up and down with round, large-holed "sieves" on their ends.

They pour regularly-changed salt water over the freshly-made butter. The Hutsuls have made dairy production into something of an artisanal handicraft, since their wooden butter and cheese forms are beautifully sculpted, while their clay pots and decoratively burnt wooden containers for milk and cream are true works of applied art. They put such heart, love, and respect into their food that it is difficult for a contemporary person to believe! Food is not a commodity but a gift of nature, which should be worshipped; it must not be sullied by a lack of effort, sloppiness, or ugliness.

Those who have spent time as guests of today's Hutsuls and have tasted their dairy say that they've never eaten anything better! Their food is all about simplicity, good energy, and kindness and boasts such a unique taste as a result! We should draw the right conclusions from such experiences, especially when we're surrounded by fast-food outlets churning out and serving millions of people their soulless, processed junk.

Remember

- Raw, unpasteurized, nonhomogenized, non-UHT dairy products, such as yogurt and kefir, are a rich source of probiotics, i.e., strains of good bacteria that are beneficial for your intestines.
- Similarly untreated full-fat butter and cream have low amounts of casein and are easily digested and assimilated.

- Cheese made from "raw" milk contains live bacteria, which have a positive effect on the digestive process.
- Pasteurized, filtered, homogenized, and UHT milk and the products made from it are best avoided.
- Milk proteins include different beta-caseins, which vary between cow breeds. There are two main categories of beta-casein, A1 and A2, each with different effects.

CHAPTER 11

SUGAR: THAT SWEET SCOUNDREL

As much as 80% of our ability to lose weight depends on what we eat. The remaining 20% is determined by our level of physical activity and other lifestyle factors.
—Mark Sisson

In many languages, words like *sweetness* and *sweet* are not only associated with certain food items but also have a range of meanings far beyond the realm of food and cooking. Delights for the palate are easily linked with complete happiness, the greatest good, a loved one, pleasantness, adoration, love, abundance, and even sexual satisfaction. Phrases like "sweet moments," "sweet nothings," "sweet dreams," "a sweet smile," "that's sweet of you," "my sweet (darling)," "sweetheart," "sweet pea," and so on are used in many different situations, cultures, and languages. At times, they also carry negative connotations of insincerity, flattery, false intentions, and crude compliments.

Like everything around us, there are two sides to sugar, which these phrases symbolically reveal. Yet, for years, people have consumed it with delight and abandon. The sweet taste of dried fruit and honey were prized by the ancient Babylonians, Egyptians, Greeks, Jews, and Romans. They considered every sweet thing to be a treat, something special, a delicacy, a delight worthy of the gods themselves.

To win Artemis's favor, the ancient Greeks left gingerbread cakes for her along their travel routes. With this same sweet and precious gift, Athenians were said to have placated a great, terrifying serpent living in a cave near their city, to ensure their safety. It wasn't just people who had a sweet tooth but the gods as well. One theory even states that the food of the gods of Mt. Olympus—nectar and ambrosia—were really honey and millet.

Although the ancient Greeks couldn't have imagined cooking without water, olive oil, milk, and honey, they consumed this last ingredient only in moderate amounts. Hippocrates of Chios (460–370 BCE) did not record a single instance of diabetes in his works. It was probably such a rare disease there would have been no sense in talking about it.

Scientists connect its later appearance at the turn of the second century CE (described by Aretaeus of Cappadocia) to the introduction of excessive amounts of honey into the diet; honey is a source of fructose, metabolized by the body into glucose. This all seems incredible considering today's diabetes problem, which is widely recognized as a social epidemic. As Dr. Mercola states, "Death by sugar may not be an overstatement: evidence is mounting that sugar is *the major factor* causing obesity and chronic disease."[141]

---

[141] Dr. Mercola, "Fructose: This Addictive Commonly Used Food Feeds Cancer Cells, Triggers Weight Gain, and Promotes Premature Aging," Mercola. com, accessed June 20, 2010, http://articles.mercola.com/sites/articles/ archive/2010/04/20/sugar-dangers.aspx.

When the words *sugar* or *sugars* appear in our discussion and in the expert's opinion just presented, we are talking about carbohydrates; the terms are synonymous. With some carbohydrates, we don't even notice a sweet taste like when we eat honey, but we're still dealing with the same molecules in pasta, kasha, bread, rice, pretzels, juice, sport drinks, and so on.

It seems most people have a cavalier attitude to eating sugar. This can even be seen among responsible mothers, who may think they're going above and beyond in their care to ensure their children's proper psychological and physical development. Each of us has probably witnessed a child's temper tantrum result in another helping of his or her favorite sweet treat.

Such a violent reaction can also be seen among addicts when first separated from the object of their addiction. Ceasing to use a substance leads to withdrawal syndrome, which can include such symptoms as irritability, aggression, anxiety, and uncontrollable behavior. As difficult as it may be to believe, *sugar is just as addictive* as heroin!

Sugar has been known to humans for a relatively short time, at least when compared to our species' evolutionary and dietary history. Like flour, sugar went into mass production only around 1850. However, it spread quickly, becoming a highly sought-after product.

It now appears in many forms: fine-grained, white, in cubes, or as a soft powder (powdered sugar). Sugar was once sold in several-kilo cones known as sugarloaves, but today, it is found in all the colors of the rainbow and in unlimited shapes and sizes, as can be seen in ready-made cake decoration sets.

Besides sugar made from sugar beets, there is also cane sugar, which comes from the exotic island of Mauritius in the Indian Ocean, among other places. This "honey-giving" cane has been known for five thousand years, but it only appeared in Europe at the height of Alexander the Great's military campaigns, when he conquered India. The product derived from sugarcane was associated with honey not just for its sweet taste but also the delicacy's amber color.

For centuries, sugar was an expensive, exclusive resource, available only to the rich and powerful. This treasure was used as a treatment for migraines and colds and as an aphrodisiac. From the Middle Ages to the latter half of the eighteenth century, it was often given as a rare gift, sometimes with entire societies pitching in to purchase it.

When we take a closer look at the figures presented in European Baroque painting, we can easily see the results of their enjoyment of this delicacy. The plump youth painted by Caravaggio (Michelangelo Merisi) and his models for *Young Bacchus* or *Amor Vincit Omnia* clearly didn't skimp on the carbs. Jusepe de Ribera's realistic works, which depict human bodies deformed by mounds of fat and bulging stomachs (e.g., *Drunken Silenus*), astonish the contemporary viewer with their grotesque obscenity.

The concept of a beautiful female figure was also no doubt shaped by a sugar-rich diet. Many of the beauties from Peter Paul Ruben's paintings are overweight, which was considered proof of their prosperity and wealth. These figures were achieved thanks to empty calories and, although they are highly sensual, are considered a bit extreme today. The paintings *The Fur* and *Angelica and the Hermit* are images of beautiful, refined, charming women, who also happen to be several pounds overweight.

Although the price of cane sugar was unusually high, the privileged classes gorged themselves on it without restraint, while their poorer subjects were not affected by this extravagant weakness. It was this period that gave rise to the well-known European saying, "The king is a great man, but even he doesn't eat sugar with a spoon."

However, cane sugar was later knocked off its pedestal by the cheaper and easier-to-produce beet sugar. Thanks to a bit of snobbism, cane sugar is still imitated by the sugar industry, as the difference in price between the two products brings a nice profit to these swindlers. They dye beet sugar with molasses or caramel color and sell it as a desirable, "organic" product. To lend credence to its exotic origin, they often warn on their labels that the product may contain traces of peanuts, sesame, soy, milk, and mustard. What a curious combination of ingredients!

The food industry quickly became interested in sugar, sensing an excellent business opportunity. It sought growing plants that could provide it. Sugarcane, sugar beets, and certain palm species began to be cultivated as a result.

Laboratories, meanwhile, soon provided synthetic substitutes, such as aspartame, and obtained corn syrup from corn. Suddenly, sugar was everywhere you looked and was even added to some surprising products: mustard, ketchup, and sauces, as well as meat and fish dishes.

So, is sugar a good old friend who, while officially here to help, is secretly conspiring against us and getting ready to deal its final blow? Will this product, a goose that lays the golden eggs in global markets, continue to be indulged by the greatest sugar and food industry concerns, regardless of the health costs to consumers?

Unfortunately, the answer to both questions is yes. For years, reliable data has clearly shown that sugar in food, in both its open and hidden forms, takes a heavy toll on human health, affecting the quality and length of our lives. Thousands of studies done by numerous independent research centers have shown that sugar is just as dangerous a toxin as cigarettes, alcohol, and heroin and that it is just as addictive.

It is the only food product that offers no nutritional value besides the energy it provides. Sugar is a source of empty calories, which are responsible for today's epidemics of high blood pressure, obesity, and diabetes. It would be impossible to get sugar approved for production today because it wouldn't pass any health tests! Everything suggests sugar would only be available on the black market at exorbitant prices.

The greatest source of empty calories in the contemporary world is sugar and more specifically high-fructose corn syrup (a mix of glucose and fructose), which is widely used in today's food industry. It is cheaper to produce than white sugar (sucrose). High-fructose corn syrup is made from corn, does not crystallize, and has a long shelf life. Despite having a disastrous effect on our health and appearance, it is everywhere in our food. It is used in sweetened beverages, candy, cookies, bread, iced tea, tonic water, energy and sports drinks, ice cream, jelly, and fruit and vegetable purees. The list goes on and on; anyone can continue compiling just by looking carefully at the labels on their food products.

I will just note that, thanks to its consistency and color, corn syrup is sometimes used as a substitute for honey in confectionery products. This glucose-fructose syrup prevents our body from releasing the hormone leptin, which is responsible for our feeling of satiety. By blocking it, corn syrup sustains a high level of ghrelin, the hunger hormone, which increases our appetite even after we've eaten a proper meal!

It's enough to look at the trends in sugar consumption over the past three hundred years.[142] The data concerns the annual sugar intake of a single person: in 1700, 4 kilograms; in 1800, 18 kilograms; in 1900, 90 kilograms; in 2009, 180 kilograms! I will just remind you that this data also covers sugar understood as refined carbohydrates: bread, pasta, dumplings, cakes, rice, juice, energy drinks, and so on. For example, one twenty-ounce bottle of Vitamin Water contains 33 grams of sugar—that's *three* Krispy Kreme original glazed doughnuts!

The expansion of sugar into human food products has been highly aggressive. Horrifyingly enough, it is even found in food for infants. Thus, our children are systematically, metabolically poisoned from the very first day they consume such products.

This shows just how little opposition there is to market forces. Neither health nor ethical concerns are enough to stop this desire for ever greater financial gain. Profit is unfortunately the priority here, relegating anything else to

---

[142] Hodan F. Well, Jean C. Buzby, "Dietary Assessment of Major Trends in US Food Consumption, 1970–2005" (PDF), *USDA Economic Research Service Economic Information Bulletin* 33 (March 2008).

the background. As they say, "Cruelty isn't such a rare human attitude at all." The lack of a decisive response to this practice works just like any learned behavior. For example, a dripping faucet is at first noticeable and irritating, but after some time, it ceases to bother us. This process of getting used to things causes us to accept a situation that is completely abnormal.

Another unpleasant (to avoid saying tragic) consequence of consuming sugar is the fact that, in 1893, not even 3 out of every 100,000 people in the United States suffered from diabetes, while today that figure has risen to 8,000 in every 100,000 citizens.[143]

You don't have to be a doctor, researcher, or statistician to see sugar's disastrous and deadly consequences. Every day, everywhere we go, we can find plenty of them. Just go to any shopping mall, peek at a school playing field, or pause by the playground to see for yourself how obesity has become the plague of civilization.

A great, uncontrollable craving for sugar can sometimes be a sign of an unhealthy and dangerous overproduction of insulin or of an addiction that is just as dangerous and difficult to fight as that of nicotine, alcohol, or narcotics. Ignoring the problem and tolerating our sweet tooth can mean unconsciously allowing these destructive processes to take place, with disastrous consequences for our health and lives. We should consider sugar to be a treacherous enemy!

---

[143] Dr. Mercola, "Fructose: This Addictive Commonly Used Food Feeds Cancer Cells, Triggers Weight Gain, and Promotes Premature Aging," Mercola. com, last updated April 20, 2010, http://articles.mercola.com/sites/articles/archive/2010/04/20/sugar-dangers.aspx.

If Caesar had been more alert to what his "loyal" comrades were up to back in 44 BCE, he likely would have avoided assassination at the hands of his close friend, Brutus. The final words of the surprised ruler were "Et tu, Brute?" The victim hadn't noticed the devious actions of his deceitful murderer in time. I mention this historical fact to warn you of your own conspiratorial enemy—sugar—so that you won't have to one day bitterly exclaim at the doctor's office, "Et tu, Brute?"

Sugars are common molecules in nature. They appear in the organic world, chiefly in plants. Sugars are made up of three elements: carbon, hydrogen, and oxygen. Hence their other name: carbohydrates. There are three types of sugar: monosaccharides (glucose, fructose), disaccharides (sucrose, maltose, lactose), and polysaccharides (starch, cellulose).

Not All Sugars Are Made Equal

The sugar most commonly found in nature is glucose, which is produced by photosynthesis in green plants. This simple sugar (monosaccharide) is sometimes called grape sugar, since the fruit contains exceptionally high amounts of it.

Our bodies convert glucose into the energy we need to live. Every cell in our body, every bacterium, and, in fact, every living being on earth uses glucose to create energy. Sugar appears in a variety of forms. Sucrose, or table sugar, is a disaccharide that is broken down into the simple sugars (monosaccharides) glucose and fructose during digestion. Glucose is the only simple sugar to appear in large amounts in our body, since all carbohydrates are converted into glucose during the digestive process.

In chemical terminology, the suffix *-ose* signifies sugar. I draw your attention to nomenclature here, since I always ask my clients (ad nauseam) to carefully read the labels on their food, even if they need a magnifying glass to do so. I hound them on it long enough for it to become ingrained in them. If any ingredient on the label ends with -ose, calmly place the item back on the shelf and ... keep looking.

Complex sugars are made up of fructose and other simple sugars. Some of them—stachyose, verbascose, and raffinose, known as oligosaccharides—occur naturally in human milk and are present in beans and other legumes. Oligosaccharides act as a soluble dietary fiber and can have a bifidogenic effect, meaning they soften stools.[144] While not yet verified as probiotics, they may promote beneficial intestinal bacteria.

Unlike herbivorous animals, humans lack the digestive enzyme necessary to break these sugars down into their simpler components. However, some people (especially those belonging to the carbohydrate metabolic type) have a certain beneficial type of flora in their large intestine that breaks down these complex sugars, producing harmless carbon dioxide in the process.

Others, unfortunately, have intestinal flora that produce foul-smelling methane, which also accompanies legume consumption. Soaking legumes in water and cooking them

---

[144] Leena Niittynen, Kajsa Kajander, Riitta Korpela, "Galacto-oligosaccharides and Bowel Function," *Scandinavian Journal of Food and Nutrition* 51 no. 2 (2007): 62–66, doi: 10.1080/17482970701414596.

for a long time makes their complex sugars easier to break down and digest. A person must have a strong, healthy, and rich intestinal microbiota to process them without a problem.

In contrast, starch (a polysaccharide made up entirely of glucose molecules) is digested and absorbed by most people. Through cooking, followed by slow and careful chewing and finally a long enzymatic process, starch is broken down into individual glucose molecules.[145]

Once in the digestive tract, glucose enters the blood through the small intestine and delivers energy to every living nook and cranny of the body, supporting all the processes taking place there, from the cellular level (e.g., thinking) to the movements of our arms and legs. One might then think, if our body transforms glucose into energy, that means sugar must be crucial to our body's functioning. But that's not true! Our fascinating bodies, perfectly shaped by evolution, can convert protein and fat into glucose—that is, into stable energy that is more potent than the energy provided by carbohydrates.

Some historically isolated ethnic groups, such as the Inuit, pre-Colombian Indians, and the medieval inhabitants of Greenland, lived almost exclusively on protein and animal fats. Studies of these people's skulls have revealed that tooth decay was foreign to them, and their teeth were virtually cavity-free. Following a nearly carbohydrate-free diet, they were distinguished by their overall good health. Unfortunately, today things look slightly different. As one article notes, "The

---

[145] By chewing, I mean grinding your food down to a nearly liquid pulp, since the enzymes in our saliva are essential for breaking down sugars.

rise in sugar intake paralleled the rise in heart disease in the Greenland Eskimo."[146]

The statistics mentioned earlier illustrate the shocking fact that only in the last century have humans begun to consume such large amounts of carbohydrates and highly processed, refined table sugar. Our ancestors, meanwhile, ate carbohydrates only seasonally, not throughout the year, and in their natural form as well (for example, fruits and vegetables).

Consumed in their ordinary state, sugar and carbohydrates come in a complete package, along with vitamins, minerals, fiber, enzymes, proteins, and fats, guaranteeing proper digestion and cellular regeneration. With such a supply of nutrients, our body is perfectly able to absorb what it needs.

Dietary fiber slows the absorption of sugar into the bloodstream, guaranteeing a healthy supply of energy, not a sugar high followed by a crash and the need for another cup of coffee. When we break this rule, the sense that we need just another cup or to somehow prop up our sleepy, drooping eyelids can linger for a while.

Most people think they know better than Mother Nature. They make fresh-squeezed orange juice, thinking that in doing so they're providing their bodies with all the vitamins and nutrients in the fruit. In fact, they're just throwing away valuable fiber.

Vitamins are not stable; most of them are damaged when exposed to air, making that glass of orange juice mere sugar

---

[146] Larry Husten, "Changes in Eskimo Diet Linked to Increase in Heart Disease," last updated July 29, 2016, http://cardiobrief.org/2016/07/29/changes-in-eskimo-diet-linked-to-increase-in-heart-disease/#comments.

water. And, by the way, the vitamin C in oranges is found in the white part of the flesh, right under the rind. Trusting Mother Nature should be the first rule of our daily diet. Fruits, vegetables, and grains, and thus carbohydrates and vitamins, only help our body function when eaten in their original form. It is only in this unprocessed state that they deliver the most valuable nutrients.

Fruit's sweetness and the flavor of fresh vegetables and grains indicate that they are ripe; full of healthy, sunshine-packed energy; and have achieved their maximum level of vitamins and minerals. The naturally sweet foods used to produce table sugar—sugar beets, sugarcane, corn, and some palms—are rich in nutrients such as vitamin B, magnesium, chromium, phosphorus, iron, calcium, and potassium. Each of these components plays an important role in controlling our blood sugar levels.

Unfortunately, they are treated as industrial waste during the sugar production process and either go unused or are added to animal feed. Refined, processed carbohydrates are unhealthy, as they have been deprived of all the elements that rebuild and heal our body, and what's more, they deplete our body's stores of vitamins, minerals, and enzymes necessary for proper metabolism.

One example of this negative effect is a vitamin B deficiency, which makes processing carbohydrates impossible. The refining process eliminates this vitamin. Quantum physicists have discovered that matter is 95 percent energy. These lifeless products steal our vitality and health like bandits, giving us nothing in return. This plunder goes unnoticed for a long time, since in the beginning it insidiously makes us feel good for a few seconds, only to later voraciously eat up our biological reserves and cause irreversible damage.

Industrial processing and refining remove the vitamins and minerals from fruits, vegetables, and grains, leaving only empty calories. Consuming refined sugar and white flour is rather like living off our savings without the habit of regularly adding to them. If we keep taking out more than we deposit, our account will eventually run dry. It's easy to see what will happen to our energy levels.

The level of glucose in our blood is regulated by an extremely delicate mechanism that uses insulin from the pancreas and other hormones from several different glands, including the adrenal glands and thyroid. When consumed in their natural form and as part of a meal containing fats and protein, sugar and starch are digested slowly, at an easy pace, and enter the bloodstream at a moderate speed over the course of several hours.

When our body goes for a longer time without food, this same mechanism uses the sugar reserves (glycogen) stored in the liver. When this marvelous regulatory process for our blood sugar levels is working properly, ensuring our cells receive a regular supply of glucose, our body is kept in perfect psychological and physical balance. However, when we consume refined sugar and starch (pizza, bread, French fries, cookies, pasta, white baked goods, juice, candy, and so on), these substances enter the blood unusually quickly, causing an unnatural spike in our blood sugar levels. At that point, our body's regulatory mechanism starts to act more like a Formula 1 driver! It hits the gas, starts running on all cylinders, and hurries to deliver insulin and other hormones to the bloodstream to quickly deal with excessive sugar levels and bring the body back into balance.

One more important note: high blood sugar levels are extremely toxic and dangerous! Sudden, repeat invasions of large amounts of sugar into the blood, like an enemy army storming into our body, cause many different types of damage to this wonderfully functioning system. Sugar opens a veritable Pandora's box of various destructive illnesses and dangerous obesity, which then threaten our system.

Completely and absolutely abstaining from refined sugar and white flour is a good idea for everyone! We must remember that these industrially produced items were practically unknown to humankind until the beginning of the seventeenth century. Yet, even then, they didn't play such a crucial and harmful role as in the twentieth century, since they were never consumed in such large amounts.

Never have they taken such a heavy toll as in today's world! Our body and its mechanisms, perfectly programmed by nature, need products in their original forms, with their entire range of undeniably valuable nutrients. Only natural products provide our bodies with the optimal sort of energy to grow and function properly. Sugar not only leads to obesity but is also responsible for many other disastrous health consequences. In addition to the increased risk of colitis and Crohn's disease, it serves as food for cancer cells and is directly linked to prostate, breast, pancreatic, lung, stomach, bladder, and gallbladder cancers.[147]

---

[147]   De Leth, OERsterk, 149.

Research done by Australian scientists shows that human genes react quite poorly to sugar consumption. It only takes two weeks of sugar in our daily diet to turn off and disable our genetic guards against diabetes and heart disease. This happens as a radical, severe reaction to a long-term, harmful diet. The process may lead to genetic damage and dysfunction that will likely be passed on to subsequent generations.

So, even if you are one of the lucky few to inherit perfect biological material from your forebears, you must still be careful and responsible when it comes to your diet. Faced with these facts, it may be hard to believe that in many Western societies, such as Poland, lovers of all things sweet are often encouraged to consume sugar with the short, cheery slogan "Sugar fortifies!"[148] When we hear something of the sort, we should stop and check whether the speaker isn't perhaps a funeral home director!

Remember

- Sugar is the main culprit behind obesity and many chronic diseases.
- The energy we absorb from protein and fats is more potent than the energy we obtain from carbohydrates.
- Sugar is just as addictive as heroin.
- Refined and highly processed carbohydrates are harmful to our body.

---

[148] Note: This is a well-known pre-World War II Polish advertising slogan—for sugar, of course. A similar sentiment might be expressed by "A spoonful of sugar helps the medicine go down."

- Eliminating refined sugar from our daily diet is the best and most sensible decision we could make for our health.
- A high-sugar diet promotes metabolic syndrome, dramatically increasing your risk for both type 2 diabetes and heart disease.

Fruit Sugar: Fructose

Fructose is a monosaccharide that appears as a simple sugar in fruit, honey, nectar, some vegetables, and flowers. It is also a component of complex sugars, e.g., sucrose (glucose + fructose), as well as raffinose and insulin. It is absorbed much more slowly by the human body than sucrose and glucose.

Fructose is a molecule commonly found in nature. It has the same molecular formula as glucose but a different structural formula. The two carbohydrates are thus isomers of one another.

From a physiological standpoint, the human intestine lacks enzymes to digest and transport fructose. Even a healthy person's capacity to absorb isolated fructose might be as little as five grams.[149]

Unfortunately, high amounts of fructose can cause diarrhea and gastrointestinal pain, and it also contributes significantly to an increase in cholesterol levels in the blood.[150] So-called low-fat diets often contain high amounts

---

[149] "Is Fructose Malabsorption a Cause of Irritable Bowel Syndrome?" accessed April 21, 2018, https://www.ncbi.nlm.nih.gov/pmc/articles/PMC4729202/.

[150] "Fructose: A Dietary Sugar in Crosstalk with Microbiota Contributing to the Development and Progression of Non-Alcoholic Liver Disease," accessed April 15, 2018, https://www.ncbi.nlm.nih.gov/pmc/articles/PMC5609573/.

of fructose. But when supplied via fruits and vegetables, fructose poses no threat to our health. Fruits, such as grapefruit, kiwifruit, and berries have relatively low fructose content and high levels of nutrients. However, fruit juices, dried fruits, and some fruits that are rich in fructose (such as pears, red apples, and plums) should be eaten relatively sparingly and in season. The research indicates that in small amounts, fructose can even help regulate the concentration of glucose in the blood.[151]

So, when does fructose consumption become a problem? The trouble starts when we have too much of it, which exceeds our body's ability to easily and thoroughly metabolize it. The entire burden of this complicated process falls to the liver, which participates in carbohydrate metabolism mainly by storing glycogen and converting galactose and fructose to grape sugar, or glucose. Two other processes also take place there: glucose production from amino acids and the formation of crucial molecules from carbohydrates and their derivatives.

Yet another strike against fructose is that, unlike other sugars, it is *"isocaloric but not isometabolic."*[152] This means you can consume the same number of calories from fructose or glucose, fructose and protein, or fructose and fat but with a completely different *metabolic effect* on your body each time—and with fructose, it's not a beneficial one.

[151] Mercola, "Clinical Scientist Sets the Record Straight on Hazards of Sugar," accessed January 20, 2015, https://articles.mercola.com/sites/articles/archive/2014/01/05/dr-johnson-leptin-resistance.aspx.
[152] Mercola, "Fructose: The Hidden Reason You Get Flabby (Not Calories or Lack of Exercise)," accessed January 20, 2015, https://articles.mercola.com/sites/articles/archive/2012/04/30/fructose-and-protein-related-to-obesity.aspx.

People today consume enormous amounts of fructose, which overloads the liver and prevents it from carrying out the processes I mentioned. The results of such a state of affairs are easy to predict; they are rather like the confusion and loss of strength we feel when we have too many obligations that all need to be met right away. A sudden increase in the consumption of carbonated drinks, sodas, or sweeteners produced from corn (corn syrup) forces our body to make an even greater destructive effort.

In the 1970s, food and beverage producers began to use corn syrup as an alternative to earlier sweeteners made from sucrose. This nearly drove cane and beet sugar off the market, since this high fructose corn syrup was discovered to be much cheaper yet 20 percent sweeter than the sugars used before. The economic (though not health) benefits turned out to be so great that they pushed scientists' warnings against this change into the background. The human body is put under unbelievable strain as it tries to deal with the huge influx of fructose from the food and drinks we consume. It must absorb it, break it down, and excrete it. Excess fructose spells metabolic disaster for our system. The effects of this destructive situation include the following:

- an increase in uric acid levels and a decrease in the level of nitric oxide, which plays a vital role in regulating the circulatory system and the functioning of the nervous system and brain[153]

---

[153] David Jockers, "Foods with Fructose: Why They're a Problem and Natural Alternatives," May 30, 2018, https://thetruthaboutcancer.com/foods-with-fructose/.

- higher levels of angiotensin, the substance that causes vasoconstriction (i.e., narrowing of the blood vessels, which increases blood pressure) and elevated blood pressure under the influence of the enzyme renin[154]
- impaired liver functioning and liver damage[155]
- a high risk of cardiovascular disease and illness due to elevated uric acid levels
- fast weight gain, which appears as abdominal obesity (a "beer belly")
- decreased HDL (good cholesterol) levels along with an increase in LDL and triglycerides[156]
- NAFLD, or nonalcoholic fatty liver disease, which is similar to the damage caused by ethanol (ethyl alcohol) metabolism[157]
- an inability to alleviate unnatural feelings of hunger, which appear because of disrupted production of the satiety hormone (leptin) and the hunger hormone (ghrelin); after consuming fructose, our hunger is

---

[154] "Fructose-rich Diet Differently Affects Angiotensin II Receptor Content in the Nucleus and a Plasma Membrane Fraction of Visceral Adipose Tissue," accessed May 30, 2018, http://www.nrcresearchpress.com/doi/abs/10.1139/apnm-2016-0725#.WxDkxmaB2i4.

[155] Mercola, "Fructose: A Dietary Sugar in Crosstalk with Microbiota Contributing to the Development and Progression of Non-Alcoholic Liver Disease," accessed April 15, 2018, https://www.ncbi.nlm.nih.gov/pmc/articles/PMC5609573/.

[156] David Jockers, "Foods with Fructose: Why They're a Problem and Natural Alternatives," May 30, 2018, https://thetruthaboutcancer.com/foods-with-fructose/.

[157] "Fructose: A Dietary Sugar in Crosstalk with Microbiota Contributing to the Development and Progression of Non-Alcoholic Liver Disease," accessed April 15, 2018, https://www.ncbi.nlm.nih.gov/pmc/articles/PMC5609573/.

still not satisfied, making fructose at least partially responsible for today's obesity epidemic[158]
- chronic vasculitis (inflammation of a blood vessel or blood vessels), which can lead to heart attack and stroke[159]

Treat your body like a temple that no garbage can defile! Desecrating this extraordinary gift of Mother Nature with just any junk food would be a true, unforgivable act of barbarism! Put yourself and your health first. As Albert Camus said, "Every minute of life carries with it its miraculous value and its face of eternal youth." [160]

Remember

- Only the small amounts of fructose provided by natural fruits and vegetables help to regulate our blood glucose level.
- Excess fructose is an absolute catastrophe that can ruin our health.
- Fructose is one of the main contributing factors behind the epidemics of obesity and cardiovascular disease.
- Avoid consuming corn syrup.

---

[158] Mercola, "Clinical Scientist Sets the Record Straight on Hazards of Sugar," accessed January 29, 2015, https://articles.mercola.com/sites/articles/archive/2014/01/05/dr-johnson-leptin-resistance.aspx.

[159] http://www.nofructose.com/introduction/.

[160] In his book, *The Sugar Fix: The High-Fructose Fallout that Is Making You Fat and Sick*, Dr. Richard Johnson shows how effective reducing your fructose consumption can be in preventing or treating chronic diseases and obesity. It also contains detailed tables of the fructose content of various food products, including fruit. His book is an invaluable resource of information that can't easily be found elsewhere. I highly recommend it!

All-Powerful Insulin

Insulin was first isolated from the pancreas in 1922. This was one of the greatest medical achievements of the twentieth century and a breakthrough in the treatment of diabetes. The anabolic peptide hormone owes its name to Jean de Mayer, who speculated in 1909 that the pancreatic islets released a substance with a hormonal effect (the Latin *insula* means island).

When the researchers Frederick Banting, Charles Best, and John Macleod used this excretion from the pancreas to treat a fourteen-year-old boy, the name proposed by Mayer turned out to be appropriate, and they adopted it as the official term. The Canadian scientists received the Nobel Prize for their discovery in 1923.

Insulin is a hormone that plays an important role mainly in the metabolism of carbohydrates but also in that of fats and protein. Carbohydrates control insulin, and insulin controls fat storage. Carbohydrates are not used as a building material by our body but are a fuel that can be burned right away by the organs and muscles or stored for later use.

All the carbohydrates we assimilate are converted into glucose in the body, which our brain, red blood cells, and nerve cells treat mainly as fuel. Less than a single teaspoon of glucose dissolved in our entire bloodstream is enough to ensure normal and safe blood sugar levels. Most healthy people's livers and muscles can store excess, unused glucose in the form of glycogen. The liver can store around 100 grams of glucose as glycogen, while the muscles can store about 500 grams,[161] though this amount depends on how fit the person is or isn't.

What happens, then, when these natural storage spaces are already full? Our body deals with this problem by converting glucose into a fatty acid and storing it in our body's fat cells. Insulin's job is to remove sugar from the blood and deposit it somewhere as quickly as possible.

It should be noted in the strongest possible terms that sugar in the blood is highly toxic! Excess carbohydrates can only be used up by those who need huge amounts of energy to play endurance sports or perform exhausting physical work. In other cases, there's no need for large amounts of carbohydrates in our diet.

The fact is carbohydrates aren't as important to our survival as protein or fats. Some scientists have estimated that the human organism can produce up to 200 grams of glucose a day from these two sources. A mere 300 grams[162] of carbohydrates eaten each day is enough to have a detrimental effect on human health. These days, some people consume several times this amount, anywhere from 500 to 600 grams![163]

Only 100 to 150 grams of carbohydrates from fruit and vegetables is enough to maintain proper insulin levels, stable energy levels, and an appropriate weight, even for those who lead a very active lifestyle. I recommend smaller amounts for overweight people, somewhere between 50 to 100 grams.

[161] Katie Vann, "How Is Excess Glucose Stored?" Livestrong.com, accessed August 16, 2013, http://www.livestrong.com/article/264767-how-is-excess-glucose-stored/. See also Hans Konrad Biesalski, Peter Grimm, *Pocket Atlas of Nutrition*, trans. Sigrid Junkermann (New York: Thieme, 2005).
[162] Sisson, *The Primal Blueprint*, 65.
[163] Ibid.

I assure you that staying within these limits is not at all difficult. As an example, a large plate of lettuce, two cups of brussels sprouts, a banana, an apple, a cup of cherries, and a cup of blueberries together give us 139 grams of carbohydrates.[164] We get such a result thanks to their valuable fiber, which is not digested and reduces the influence of glucose concentrations in the blood. I would like to note here that it is not a good idea to make fruit or vegetable juices and just throw this valuable fiber away.

Diabetes—The Twenty-First Century's Health-Related Leviathan

I strongly believe that the more we know about health and the relationship between our bodies and what we eat, the more empowered we are to live healthy, happy, fulfilling lives. When we understand how our bodies work—what is actually going on when we ingest certain foods and make lifestyle choices—it is like one of those great aha moments in life. It's that sense of "Now, I get it. I can see why I feel this way, have these health problems, or face these health obstacles."

On a collective level, it is precisely these basic misunderstandings and gaps in our knowledge base that are behind many of the global health epidemics that we are facing today. Nowhere is this more evident than with insulin resistance and the monumental numbers of people suffering from diabetes and obesity, as well as the complications that result from these health conditions.

---

[164] Sisson, *The Primal Blueprint*, 89.

In the United States, sixty to seventy million people suffer from insulin resistance,[165] with around ten million in Poland and thirty-five million in Russia also suffering from the condition.[166] Statistics show that the situation is not much better in other countries. It has been predicted that over 40 percent of people aged fifty or over may be at risk of insulin resistance. This condition, however, can occur at any age.[167]

What is going on with insulin and the modern human body? Why is it that, in this era, we are facing such a formidable obstacle to well-being? Diabetes has become the twenty-first century's health-related leviathan. It's huge. It's ruining lives, taking lives in some cases, and is causing health-care professionals around the world to throw their hands up in the air, unable to cure a disease that's incurable. It is incurable because we are doing it to ourselves. Yes, it is true that age and genetics can increase your risk of becoming a diabetic. Slightly. In some cases, insulin resistance can be caused by factors such as *polycystic ovary syndrome*, which, while it affects your diet and the way your body processes

---

[165] National Diabetes Fact Sheet, 2011, Centers for Disease Control, accessed August 29, 2012, www.cdc.gov/diabetes/pubs/pdf/ndfs_2011.pdf. See also Yvette C. Terrie, "Insulin Resistance: Recognizing the Hidden Danger," *Pharmacy Times*, October 5, 2012, http://www.pharmacytimes.com/publications/issue/2012/October2012/Insulin-Resistance-Recognizing-the-Hidden-Danger.

[166] "Statistics by Country for Insulin Resistance," from the US Census Bureau, International Data Base, 2004, Rightdiagnosis.com, Health Grades Inc., last updated August 13, 2015, http://www.rightdiagnosis.com/i/insulin_resistance/stats-country.htm.

[167] "About Diabetes," American Heart Association, accessed August 29, 2012, www.heart.org/HEARTORG/Conditions/Diabetes/AboutDiabetes/AboutDiabetes_UCM_002032_Article.jsp.
See also "Insulin Resistance: Recognizing the Hidden Danger."

sugar, is not caused by diet. Type 1 diabetes, for instance, is theorized to be genetic.

The reality is that most of the cases are primarily due to a combination of a sedentary lifestyle and poor eating habits; genetic predisposition is just the icing on the cake that leads to insulin resistance.

While this reality may seem harsh, it is only through accepting our own responsibility for our health that we can, as individuals and as a society, take back control of our well-being.

Right now, there is such a need for clear, accurate information on the subject of insulin resistance, what's causing it, and what can be done about it. Much of the public information available today, even directly from the medical community, is extremely nearsighted, outdated, and disempowering. Real guidance is also hard to come by.

Past health campaigns may have been well-meaning, but they have also served the purpose of diluting and confusing our knowledge of how the body metabolizes food and have, to an extent, caused our diets to change in such a way that has contributed to the shocking prevalence of diabetes today. For example, the belief that all fats are "bad" and anything "low-fat" is good is one of the largest health untruths of all time. It is an inaccuracy that has led to a cascade of disastrous health decisions for decades, like shunning whole, nourishing foods like avocados, nuts, and seeds and instead, grabbing the processed, packaged, often high-sugar "low-fat" items off the grocery shelves. Food manufacturers, of course, capitalized on these myopic health messages with multi-million-dollar marketing campaigns touting the benefits of foods that have proved to be more of a problem than a solution.

I truly believe that most people want to feel healthy and would make better choices if they had access to the right information. When it comes to insulin, a clear understanding of what this hormone does and how much our bodies need is essential to ensuring we aren't walking on a path toward insulin resistance and a whole sea of health problems. Once you know the role that insulin plays and how to best support this hormone to do its job properly, you have taken a giant leap toward better health.

Insulin's Goal Is Balance

Insulin is one of those things that we need but only in very small amounts. Too much, and it becomes harmful rather than helpful. You may know that insulin regulates your blood sugar levels, but it does much more than this.

Insulin is a peptide hormone that is used to store sugars as fat. This is why when we eat more carbohydrates, our pancreas produces more insulin. It is basically trying to cope with the high blood sugar levels. This hormone also delivers sugar, as well as nutrients, to cells, to keep them functioning properly.

Insulin's role is often likened to that of a key. When this system works according to our body's natural evolutionary blueprint, the cells' receptors use insulin like a key to unlock pores in the membrane of each cell. These openings allow the needed components, namely sugar and nutrients, to enter. It's truly an amazing process, as everything that needs to enter each cell does, while at the same time excess glucose is removed and stored for later use as glycogen in the liver, which prevents a toxic buildup from occurring.

This is how the system has evolved to work according to how our bodies consume food. The problem is that when overworked, the pancreas stops functioning properly and will start producing excess insulin. The modern diet consists of lots of carbohydrates, processed foods, and sugars. When combined with a sedentary lifestyle, this puts too much pressure on the pancreas.

Years of consuming excess carbohydrates and failing to eat a balanced diet can start to move this quite delicate system off-track. Once the pancreas starts producing too much insulin, the problem can rapidly spiral out of control.

First, the muscles and liver are not able to take in and store the excess buildup of glycogen—the substance insulin converts glucose to. This means there is now even more glucose in the blood. What happens to it?

Some of this excess glucose can be used up by your muscle cells when you engage in intense exercise or your brain cells when you engage in intellectual work. The rest is converted into triglycerides in the liver, which is then transported to your fat cells for storage.

If that wasn't enough, as the levels of insulin in the blood are high, the fat cells that normally store excess glucose also store fat from every meal that you consume. At this point, the insulin is telling these fat cells to hold on to everything. The elegant system that partitioned food to be used as energy and stored for later use is now storing everything. Nothing is being burned off and converted into energy.

Imagine what is happening to these poor fat cells. Naturally, once this process is repeated, the fat cells begin to swell. This is where people start to put on weight quickly. Also, both the muscle and liver cells have become resistant to insulin. This often occurs when people are not physically active. This means your body has far bigger problems than weight gain. The cells' receptors are not responding to signals described earlier that insulin sends out—instructing cells to unlock their membranes to allow nutrients to enter. This is what many people don't realize. Obesity is, in truth, a sign of serious nutritional deficiencies.

This cascading negative effect doesn't stop here. Keep in mind that fat also performs a protective function for our body. Our bodies' fat cells intercept and accumulate toxins so they can be burned off later and removed from our body, rather than flowing through our bloodstream and, over time, causing us harm. There are two hundred times more toxins in our fat cells than in our bloodstream![168]

The more overweight someone is, the more toxins his or her fat tissue contains. More fat storage in a body that is insulin resistant is equal to more toxins poisoning our bodies and fewer nutrients supporting our health. Now you see why diabetes and obesity epidemics are causing a very complex global health crisis. This simple imbalance opens up the body for so many more diseases, in addition to an overall sense of fatigue, lethargy, and sickness rather than one of vitality, strength, and well-being.

---

[168] Nan Kathryn Fuchs, "How to Protect Yourself from the Harmful Effects of Toxins," accessed June 20, 2015, https://www.bewellbuzz.com/email/bwb78.html.

Toxic glucose in the blood and impaired insulin production can lead to diabetes, heart disease, and many other illnesses. High insulin levels can contribute to cancer growth, as cancer feeds on glucose (carbohydrates). This fuel is provided by insulin.

As the liver becomes insulin resistant because of a system that has become, quite literally, unchecked, things get even worse. One would assume that the liver would take in the extra glucose, but what happens is that it is not absorbed. The liver cells are tricked into thinking they are deficient in glucose. This triggers a reaction called gluconeogenesis, which is the conversion of nonsugar elements into sugar, e.g., more fatty acids. Yet another load of sugar goes into the bloodstream, where there's already plenty. Guess where this batch of excess sugar goes?

You guessed it. This completely new load of glucose from the liver goes straight to the fat cells. One only hopes those already overloaded cells can handle it!

That's the End of the Damage, Right?

Unfortunately, no! Insulin has proinflammatory properties that can wreak havoc throughout the body. This damage may not be immediately apparent. In fact, most of it happens gradually. We may not be aware of it until our health has deteriorated to a point of no return.

Scientists proved long ago that the longest-living mammals were those that produced the least insulin. High levels of insulin in the blood are a fundamental contributing factor in the development of coronary heart disease. Insulin affects platelet adhesion, causing these cells to stick to the walls of our blood vessels more quickly and easily. It is also responsible for changing white blood cells into foam cells—these are the white blood cells that have combined with cholesterol. They accumulate along our artery walls, causing hardening and thinning. Insulin also reduces nitric oxide, a substance known to increase blood flow and prevent sticky plaque from building up and hardening the arteries, thereby further exacerbating this atherosclerotic state.

There is nothing pleasant about this negative cycle of insulin resistance caused by a diet high in refined sugar and simple carbohydrates, yet it is entirely preventable and in many cases, reversible. What is necessary is for more people to understand how important it is to get enough physical activity and to eat the right diet. What's the right diet for healthy insulin levels? A low-carb diet without any refined sugar but lots of fresh vegetables and fruits, organic protein, and fats. It's also important to get enough sleep and to proactively manage stress. There is another relationship that should be noted here: high levels of cortisol—the stress hormone—correspond to high insulin levels.

This is really fascinating as well. High levels of insulin have a negative impact on human growth hormones as well as other hormones, such as the youth hormone DHEA, testosterone, and others. Therefore, insulin also affects the functioning of the pituitary gland and thyroid, which produces the T4 hormone that is converted into T3 in the liver. When the liver demonstrates insulin resistance, this conversion of T4 to T3 is drastically reduced, resulting in a slowed-down metabolism and fat buildup.[169]

What does this mean? This is an exponential process. Impaired insulin regulation leads to weight gain, toxin buildup, nutritional deficiencies, hardening of the arteries, and even a huge obstacle to turning things around, as your metabolism is slower, your body has developed a system of fat storage, and the energy and even mental will to exercise and eat well may be difficult to muster—at first. But this is a process that can go both ways. You choose the direction. Every step toward healthier insulin levels as a result of healthy eating habits and exercise makes the next and then the next step toward well-being that much easier.

Of course, it is not always a person's fault when he or she gets fatal and debilitating diseases and disorders caused by genetics, like, for example, Huntington's chorea and cystic fibrosis. But single-gene disorders (when a certain gene is known to cause a disease) affect less than 2 percent of the population.[170] Bruce Lipton in his book *The Biology of Belief* stated, "The diseases that are today's scourges—diabetes, heart diseases, and cancer—short-circuit a happy and healthy life. These diseases, however, are not the result of a single gene, but of the complex interaction among multiple genes and environmental factors."[171] It means that most of us come into this world with genes that allow us to live a happy and healthy life.

---

[169] Gabriela Brenta, "Why Can Insulin Resistance Be a Natural Consequence of Thyroid Dysfunction?" *Journal of Thyroid Research*, vol. 2011, Article ID 152850, 9 pages (2011), doi:10.4061/2011/152850.

[170] Lipton, *The Biology of Belief,* 21.

[171] Lipton, *The Biology of Belief,* 21.

"What about a Little Something? … Well, I Shouldn't Mind a Little Something!"

It may be tempting to believe "a little something" won't affect us at all, but nothing could be further from the truth. Any time we eat a product high in carbohydrates, our blood glucose levels go shooting up and affect our mood, energy levels, concentration, and alertness. In the space of only a few minutes (depending on what kind of carbohydrates we've eaten), insulin rushes to lower our sugar levels so quickly that our glucose-dependent brain is left almost without fuel. We experience this in the form of fatigue, moodiness, indecisiveness, and even aggression and distraction. This process also explains our need for an afternoon nap. Let's take a closer look at the stages of this phenomenon:

1. You feel tired, but you've still got a million things to do.
2. You decide to consume more sugar, coffee, tea, and refined carbohydrates, such as breakfast cereal, bread, a candy bar, jam, Jell-O, cookies, or some other snack.
3. Your blood sugar level rises after you drink another coffee and absorb some refined carbohydrates.
4. With this rise in blood sugar, and following the jolt you get from another serving of caffeine, stress hormones are released as part of a fight-or-flight response. This starts up many chemical processes that lead to the creation of glycogen, the form of sugar stored in the liver, which is then converted into glucose and enters

the bloodstream, so that you can "fight or flee" more quickly.

5. Now you're literally swimming in sugar! Insulin must be sent in to help, so that all this sugar can be stored away and hidden before it ends up damaging our nerve cells or other tissues. Insulin must hurry, and when it finishes its work, you feel tired, irritated, and hungry.

6. This drop in energy and new feelings of hunger are usually signs that the process is about to start all over again!

This is clearly a vicious cycle. These stages are accompanied by other, short-lived symptoms, which may include fat accumulation around the navel (this fat then spreads to other parts of the body), neck and shoulder pain, lower back pain, a suppressed immune system, mood swings, difficulty concentrating, and low energy levels.

We should pay particular attention to the way sugar inhibits our immune system. Sugar is tied to unstable energy levels and stress. In turn, chronic production of the stress hormone cortisol severely hampers immune function.

Scientists have also shown that sugar can impair the functioning of the cells in our immune system—phagocytes—that remove bacteria and viruses from the blood. Sugar's impact lingers for up to five hours after we've ingested it.[172] This leads to the phenomenon known as competitive inhibition, in which vitamin C is unable to enter cells in the presence of excess glucose. This is because both molecules use the same system to get inside the cell. As a result, this process creates

---

[172]   Sisson, *The Primal Blueprint*, 72.

the ideal conditions for harmful free radicals to flourish. The chain of events presented here happens even in people who are healthy (for now) and who regularly consume excess amounts of carbohydrates and refined sugar.

***

This "sweet scoundrel" is always half a step behind us, ready to pounce when we least expect it and ruin our health and lives in a variety of ways. Unfortunately, most of its destructive effects are irreversible, even tragic. Take a moment to think first, and then ... slowly draw your hand away from the sugar bowl, filled to the brim with a white substance *whose reputation is anything but crystal clear*. As the old Polish folk saying goes "There's no sweet without the bitter."

How is it possible that so many of us still consume so much sugar? How is this highly dangerous substance still in everyday use? I don't wish to frighten you into permanent suspicion of anything and everything you find on your plate. Rather, I'd like to arm you with the right informational weapons to fight sugar's insidious, damaging effects, allowing you to limit its presence in your daily diet.

Remember

- Carbohydrates control insulin, and insulin controls fat storage.
- Our body does not use carbohydrates as a building material.

- Less than a single teaspoon of glucose dissolved in our entire bloodstream is enough to ensure normal and safe blood sugar levels.
- A mere 300 grams of carbohydrates eaten each day are enough to harm human health.
- Our insulin levels are of fundamental importance to our health and lives.
- People who are not physically active are at risk of developing insulin-resistant muscle and liver cells.
- Insulin has pro-inflammatory properties and can wreak havoc throughout the entire body.
- The presence of high levels of insulin in the blood is a fundamental contributing factor in the development of coronary heart disease.
- A waist circumference of over 35 inches (90 centimeters) in women and 40 inches (100 centimeters) in men is one indication of insulin resistance.

CHAPTER 12

THE MINCED TRUTH ABOUT WHOLE-GRAIN FOOD

Nobody is qualified to become a statesman who
is entirely ignorant of the problem of wheat.
—Socrates

For many years, I've observed our mainstream eating habits change with calm detachment. Every so often—like chaos tearing apart the existing order—a new trend comes along and causes utter mayhem in consumers' daily diets.

At social functions, when talking with friends or when gathered around the holiday table, the topic of food occasionally comes up. Listening to the resulting discussions is fascinating, as they reveal such a diversity of views as traditional attitudes clash with new, opposing ideas.

One hears a litany of rational justifications and assurances: "That's healthy," "I won't touch that," "That's worked for me for years," and so on. When counterarguments are made, they come with a healthy dose of instinctive defense mechanisms and self-limiting beliefs and convictions. In short, discord reigns. Curiously, even among the highly educated, you can see a certain amount of confusion in this area and in many cases simple ignorance.

Most of society is drowning in this ocean of uncertainty, since the all-encompassing conventional wisdom can lead even the sharpest and best minds astray. So, today one of the main questions that you can hear is what about bread?

Grains in History

When they imagined the origins of the world, the ancient Greeks said that first there was *chaos*. Nobody, however, could say exactly what that chaos was. Some considered it to be a divine being but without a concrete form, while others believed it was a gaping emptiness, a great abyss, a black void preceding the creation of the world.

They eventually concluded that *chaos* is a special substance full of creative power, the divine seeds and origins of everything, all blended together with the four elements of earth, water, fire, and air. This chaos contained the beginnings of the future world and the Cosmos, Gaia, and Uranus.

The Greeks worshipped seeds, as they symbolized the gift of life, fertility, abundance, existence, and everything needed to live. Just as revered were grains. A core part of our ancestors' diets, ancient peoples from the Romans to the Egyptians and the Mayans valued grains for their life-giving sustenance. They were viewed as more than mere food but a force for supporting life and civilization.

In many cultures, bread, cakes, and other simple baked goods were staple foods. Excavations have allowed us to date their use by humankind back to more or less twelve thousand years ago. The flour or meal obtained from the crushed grains was used to make cakes from batter poured onto flat, heated stones. The Egyptians were likely the first to use fermentation to raise baked goods. The ancient Romans also attributed special significance to grains, using freshly ground flour, meal, and water to make cakes that newly married couples would eat in the presence of ten witnesses to validate their marriage. They also sprinkled grains over sacrificial animals before killing them.

It is easy to see that, throughout human history, grains have played many culinary, religious, magical, and symbolic roles. Of course, they are still present in the diet of contemporary humans, but today they are a subject of controversy among professionals and laypeople alike. Some argue that whole-grain products have always been found in our daily diet. Their honest intentions and the advice of dieticians to consume whole-grain products like our ancestors are misleading and often harmful.

Our prehistoric forebears obviously ate whole-grain foods but not in the way that today's cookbooks or diets recommend and certainly not in an industrially processed form. It seems they first soaked the grains or allowed them to ferment, only then making bread from them or grinding them into groats. Such actions reveal our ancestors' great wisdom and complete trust in Mother Nature.

Before they began to use stone tools to grind cereals, they observed how the plant naturally protected these grains against destruction. After all, a grain is unable to fight or flee. Multiple hard layers of chaff or shells effectively resisted any attempt to damage their contents. Living in harmony with nature and demonstrating unusual humility in the face of its mechanisms and strength, our ancestors saw how well this strong, tight outer coating worked in inhospitable habitats, in frozen soil, or during drought.

Today, we can add one more note to their observations: plant seeds contain antinutrients (pectins, saponins, gluten, and phytic acid), which hamper our body's ability to absorb important molecules and vitamins. These antinutrients are meant to protect the seed from harmful microorganisms and pathogens.

Seeds also accumulate the remains of heavy metals, which form a sort of barrier that makes it impossible for these dangerous organisms to get inside. They also provide protection against the chemicals commonly used in farming. When consuming the seeds of yew or mistletoe, for example, many bird species do not digest them; instead, they excrete them somewhere else (a clever evolutionary method of plant propagation).

Grains, which contain protein, carbohydrates, fats, and vitamins, are the ideal food for many species of mycotoxin-producing fungi, which are also incredibly hazardous to our health. We won't speculate here about what mysterious spirit inspired our ancestors to soak and ferment grains before eating them. It seems simple when we try to bite into a hard, dry grain of wheat or rye and see how much effort is needed to transform it into a swallowable pulp.

Having likely tried something similar themselves, our ancestors began not only to soften grains in water but also pour them between two flat stones to grind them down, thus saving their teeth. Turning their hand-operated millstones, known as querns, required long and persistent effort, thanks to which our forebears also built up their physical fitness. Today's scientists have discovered these methods and confirmed their usefulness. But what humankind had always intuitively known to be correct has been forgotten and eliminated today, and grains are now soaked and fermented most effectively by the alcohol industry!

The Staff of Life—Bread

In many cultures, independently and regardless of their geographical region, bread is not only an ordinary, everyday food but also a traditional staple of human subsistence.

In the book of Ecclesiasticus, bread is one of the "chief things for life," along with water, clothing, and a house, while the popular Christian Lord's Prayer includes a request to God to give us our daily bread. The consumption of bread takes on a ceremonial and symbolic character in many religions, where bread is a sacred object of worship.

For example, the figure of Christ is found in the form of "bread and wine" in the Christian Eucharist. He introduces himself to his followers with the words, "I am the bread of life." Eating bread is practically a religious imperative and respect for it a solemn duty. In many societies, bread is never thrown away, and if it falls to the ground, it is picked up and kissed. Until recently, people in Poland would make the sign of the cross over a loaf before slicing it, and to this day, the parents of newlyweds greet their children at the reception venue with bread and salt.

But is this ancient bread the same as today's? Could we cry out enthusiastically for "bread and circuses" (*panem et circenses*) like the ancient Romans did? Would the white, unleavened bread of the Israelites be accepted without concern by today's dieticians? These are difficult questions to answer conclusively, since wheat, from which most ancient bread was made, has been known to humankind for thousands of years and is one of the oldest bread-making cereals.

Today, there are around twenty varieties of wheat, but none of them is the grain that our ancestors consumed. Today's consumers must contend with dwarf wheat—the product of genetic manipulation and cross-breeding—and not the well-known heirloom varieties like single-grain Einkorn or double-grain Emmer wheat, which have been cultivated since at least 7000 to 8000 BCE.

Today's varieties are extremely high-yield plants,[173] with higher levels of starch and gluten and many more chromosomes than what our ancestors ate. The man who developed this new, modified strain of wheat received the Nobel Prize for his work and promised to feed the hungry around the world. However, this attempt to improve upon Mother Nature has led to the obesity of millions of people and has instead become proof of humankind's irresponsible, careless ignorance and vanity.

The primary difference between contemporary and ancient wheat is that today's wheat contains high amounts of a starch known as amylopectin A. Two slices of bread made from this

---

[173] It's factory farming for plants.

wheat raises our blood sugar more than two tablespoons of table sugar.[174] This is definitely bad news for our pancreas!

Ancient grains contained fourteen chromosomes and caused health problems even then, if not prepared properly. Today's hybrids have twenty-eight chromosomes and produce a wide variety of gluten proteins, which cause our body to react in new, harmful ways.[175] They are impossible to digest.

What's more, there's no difference between white flour and whole-wheat products. The greatest scam perpetrated on the public by food producers, who allegedly care about our health, is their practice of including the term "whole-grain" on food labels as a way of making themselves seem more virtuous and caring. Many processed foods full of sugar, cheap fats, and wheat flour are advertised as being organic and whole-grain.

The Mass Production Problem

Just as detrimental to our health is the actual process used to make our bread. Think of the bread our ancestors ate—made from pure strains of the grain, no genetic modifications, all grown in chemical-free fields of golden wheat, and then prepared by hand with zero additives, allowed to slowly rise, and baked in a wood-fired hearth.

Compare that to what goes on today in industrial bread manufacturing, and you can see why so many people are having trouble digesting food, let along enjoying it, and many

---

[174] Mark Hyman, "Three Hidden Ways Wheat Makes You Fat," *Huffington Post*, February 18, 2012, http://www.huffingtonpost.com/dr-mark-hyman/wheat-gluten_b_1274872.html.

[175] Ibid.

are experiencing adverse health effects ranging from minor to severe.

Thanks to a process developed in 1961 by scientists at the Chorleywood Flour Milling and Bakery Research Association Laboratories based in southern England,[176] bread can be produced quickly and at scale. It takes about three and a half hours to go from raw ingredients to a loaf of packaged bread, ready to be shipped to sit on the shelves in the grocery store for consumers to purchase.

No more long fermentation process, as the yeast is allowed to do its work, causing the dough to rise and getting that great, fluffy texture. No more worries about loaves going moldy or drying out and losing their squishy texture after a few days—like any normal homemade loaf of bread would do.

Think about it. You can buy packaged bread at the store and expect to keep it on your kitchen counter or in the refrigerator to eat for a week or two. Even though it could have been made days, maybe a week or more, before you even bought it and took it home. But it will still be soft and mold-free.

This is excellent news for bread producers, but what it takes to create this convenience is really bad news for your health. In order to create this cheap, long-shelf-life bread, producers have to use a lot of additives to get the right texture and to preserve the bread while it sits for days—or weeks. These additives could be behind a lot of the health problems people are experiencing from eating bread, like the digestive and skin issues, difficulty losing weight, and low energy levels.

---

176 Barbara Griggs, "The Rise and Rise of Sourdough Bread," accessed April 15, 2018, https://www.theguardian.com/lifeandstyle/2014/aug/12/rise-sourdough-bread-slow-fermented-health-benefits.

Because guess what industrial bread producers are loading our sandwich slices and morning toast with? Yep—extra gluten.

They add extra gluten as well as other additives like processed fats for texture, soy flour to increase volume, emulsifiers, preservatives, and lots of extra yeast for a super-fast rise without the actual fermentation that helps to deactivate the natural gluten in the first place.

The question we really need to look at is this: Are people getting sick from the bread they eat because they are just sensitive and can't tolerate the additives—or are people developing an intolerance because they are eating industrially processed bread?

A few years ago, a study published in the journal *Gastroenterology* that looked at indicators for celiac disease in the blood found that the presence of these indicators has increased by 400 percent in the past fifty years.[177] Even if you don't have celiac, the chance of facing health problems from a wheat intolerance is something we all should be concerned about.

Health-care practitioners and nutritionists are seeing a rise in the number of patients with gluten or wheat intolerance. Nutrition therapist and yoga instructor Lisa Christie was quoted in the *Guardian* saying, "Gluten sensitivity is one of the most common problems I see in my practice. Ditching commercial breads is a great step for anyone to improve health and wellbeing, and for many of my patients, restricting their gluten intake to properly-made sourdough bread—wholegrain wheat, rye, emmer or kamut—works really well." [178]

---

[177]   Ibid.
[178]   Ibid.

Sourdough Health Solution

In the traditional preparation of sourdough bread, however, the gluten is naturally modified during the slow fermentation process. The bread rises gradually, which yields a type of bread our bodies can digest and can actually benefit from nutritionally because gluten and other additives aren't wreaking havoc on our gut.

If you make sourdough yourself or buy sourdough bread freshly made from your local bakery, especially if they use a pure type of wheat like Einkorn, you won't have all those troubling additives. But what you will have is a bread that is rich in antioxidants, B vitamins, folic acid, and important minerals like iron, zinc, and magnesium—key minerals that the typical Western diet is deficient in.

Studies have also found that sourdough made with slow fermentation produces a lower glucose and insulin response, making it a healthier alternative for diabetics.

To bake sourdough bread, all you need is organic flour, water, and salt—none of the unnatural ingredients found in commercial bread. Cheap, industrially produced bread always comes with all those chemical additives you shouldn't be putting in your body, and that is behind the prevalence of wheat intolerances today. Sourdough bread is made using only wild yeast.[179] Wild yeast needs a little more coaxing and works a little more slowly than commercial yeast, so

---

[179] Vanessa Kimbell, "Why Is It that I Can Digest Sourdough Bread and Not Commercial Bread?" *The Sourdough School*, last updated January 21, 2017, http://www.sourdough.co.uk/why-is-it-that-i-can-digest-sourdough-bread-and-not-commercial-bread/.

sourdough breads are normally mixed, shaped, and baked over the course of an entire day, even multiple days.

While wild yeast is certainly the star of this show, it's not actually the yeast that makes the bread "sour" and easy for us to assimilate and digest. That job is done by friendly bacteria—*Lactobacillus*, cousins of the bacteria that curdle milk into yogurt and cheese—which grow alongside the wild yeast in the sourdough culture, helping to ferment the sugars in the dough and predigest gluten. The wild yeast and *Lactobacillus* neutralize the phytic acid in the dough, making the resulting bread easier to digest. Removing phytic acid is key; otherwise, the acid binds with minerals, such as calcium, magnesium, iron, and zinc, making them unavailable. Long, slow wheat fermentation can reduce up to 90 percent of the phytic acid.[180] The lactic acid bacteria present in sourdough enhances acidification, leading to greater magnesium and phosphorus solubility.[181] So, you get a delicious bread that nourishes instead of harming your body.

The Thief Who Should Be Drowned!

Phytic Acid

All grains, bran, beans, seeds, and nuts contain phytic acid (phytates), which is a common chemical in the plant world, particularly in cereal grains. The chief concern about phytic acid is that it can bind to certain dietary minerals, including

---

[180]   Ibid.
[181]   Ibid.

iron, zinc, manganese, and, to a lesser extent, calcium, and block their absorption.

Phytic acid (phytates) became a problem in our diet when we lost contact with the traditions of our ancestors who could prepare grains for consumption quite well.

Phytic acid (phytates) is a thief that steals essential resources from our system. Osteoporosis, rickets, and anemia became common diseases even among the first farmers. In the Middle Ages, when yeast began to be widely used as a bread leavening agent, rickets became a societal plague.

Unlike with a sourdough starter, the presence of yeast does not neutralize the thieving effects of phytic acid. The spread of grain cultivation, centuries of poverty among a large part of Europe's population, and high meat prices encouraged a plain, unvaried diet, resulting in malnourishment and the appearance of rickets in 80 percent of Northern European children even as late as the nineteenth century.[182]

Only by soaking grains do we enable enzymes and other helpful microorganisms to break down and neutralize phytates as well as predigest gluten. Leaving them to soak for a few hours[183] in warm water with sea salt or with an acidic medium added, e.g., whey (or yogurt), neutralizes the negative properties of phytic acid. What little acid is left helps protect against cancer, since in such small amounts, this acid does, in fact, have a beneficial effect. It also may help prevent cardiovascular disease.[184]

---

[182] *Wikipedia*, The Free Encyclopedia, s.v., "Kwas Fitowy [Phytic Acid]," http://pl.wikipedia.org/wiki/Kwas_fitowy.

[183] Seventy-five percent of the phytate is broken up within ten hours.

[184] Andrew Weil, "Are Phytates Bad or Good?" accessed May 2, 2017, https://www.drweil.com/diet-nutrition/nutrition/are-phytates-bad-or-good/.

This "submersion" attack pacifies the pillaging acid and also boosts the nutritional properties of the grains to be eaten. In their whole form, grains play a big role in blocking the metabolism of vitamin D and contribute to vitamin C and B12 deficiencies. Scientists have found that proteins from certain seeds (as well as from some dairy products) imitate the proteins found in viruses and bacteria, thus tricking our immune system.[185]

Gluten

Gluten is a protein substance found in the grains of nearly all cereal crops. This large, water-soluble mix of proteins is what makes dough elastic and sticky (these properties are also why it's used to produce wallpaper adhesive). These proteins are very difficult to digest. They are found in the highest amounts in wheat, which (besides rice) is humankind's most important and widespread food crop. Scientists consider gluten to be the cause of many allergies, celiac disease, some psychological disorders, chronic indigestion, digestive system disorders, mycosis, dermatitis, joint pain, fertility problems, hyperacidity, acid reflux, and autoimmune diseases.[186]

Grains are divided into two categories: those that contain gluten (wheat, rye, barley, oats) and gluten-free grains (buckwheat, rice, millet). The former should be consumed

---

[185] William Davis, *Wheat Belly Total Health*, 273.

[186] Anna Sapone, Julio C. Bai, Carolina Ciacci, Jernej Dolinsek, Peter H. R. Green, Marios Hadjivassiliou, Katri Kaukinen, Kamran Rostami, David S. Sanders, Michael Schumann, Reiner Ullrich, Danilo Villalta, Umberto Volta, Carlo Catassi, and Alessio Fasano, *Spectrum of Gluten-Related Disorders: Consensus on New Nomenclature and Classification*, accessed June 8, 2018, https://www.ncbi.nlm.nih.gov/pmc/articles/PMC3292448/.

after being soaked or fermented, while the latter are easily digested and contain low levels of phytic acid.

Wholegrain rice and millet should be cooked for at least two hours in a gelatin-rich, homemade broth. That way, the phytates are neutralized, while the gelatin from the bones makes them easier to digest.

Gluten also contains addictive substances, just like sugar. Once processed by our digestive system, these proteins are transformed into shorter polypeptides, called exorphins. They are similar to the endorphins our body creates when running, for example, or when needed to relieve pain or suffering. This phenomenon was studied and first described as a "runner's high" in the 1970s. The opioid receptors in the brain are sensitive to these endorphins, as well as many other substances provided by the food or medicines we consume. These compounds have proven opioid effects and could mask the deleterious effects of gluten protein on gastrointestinal function and lining. Here, we describe a putative mechanism, explaining how gluten could "mask" its own toxicity by exorphins that are produced through gluten protein digestion.[187]

The plant world is full of various defense mechanisms to protect plants' seeds from damage and scare off potential enemies. Many plants have thorns, hard coatings, or a repulsive odor. Many also contain poisonous, paralyzing, or sleep-inducing compounds. Wheat contains this last type of substance and, with the help of opioid peptides, is able to

---

[187]   L. Pruimboom and K. de Punder, *The Opioid Effects of Gluten Exorphins: Asymptomatic Celiac Disease*, accessed June 8, 2018, https://www.ncbi.nlm.nih.gov/pubmed/26825414.

defend itself against complete annihilation. These are known as gluteomorphins (after "gluten" and "morphine").

Their properties were known even among the earliest civilizations. Ancient Egyptian priests used them for medicinal and magical purposes. Wheat was used to relieve pain related to rheumatism, broken bones, and other injuries. It was also used to induce hallucinations, which the Egyptians believed encased important prophecies.

Gluteomorphins are the cause of addictive eating behavior, including cravings and bingeing. And they can also cause multiple problems, including schizophrenia and autism.[188] Wheat gluten contains extremely addictive opioid peptides. Some of these peptides can be one hundred times stronger than morphine. In plain language, *wheat is an addictive appetite stimulant.*

One other problem is gliadins, a glycoprotein that is also another component of gluten. Research by Alessio Fasano, MD, of the University of Maryland School of Medicine suggests gliadin causes zonulin levels in the intestines to increase. As a result, the seal between the intestinal cells diminishes, opening up spaces between cells that allow all sorts of things to pass right through. This occurs in people who have celiac disease and those who do not; for anyone, chronic exposure to gluten can harm the gut.[189] But the good

[188] Mark Hayman, *Three Hidden Ways Wheat Makes You Fat*, accessed June 8, 2018, https://www.huffingtonpost.com/dr-mark-hyman/wheat-gluten_b_1274872.html?guccounter=1.

[189] Alessio Fasano, "Zonulin, Regulation of Tight Junctions, and Autoimmune Diseases," accessed June 18, 2017, https://www.ncbi.nlm.nih.gov/pmc/articles/PMC3384703/.

news is removing gluten from the diet can resolve and reverse the problem quite quickly.

Lectins

Besides phytates and gluten, cereal grains and many other plants contain the plant toxins known as lectins. Scientists have discovered that these compounds hamper digestive function and damage the delicate lining of the intestines. They can easily transform our intestines into a leaky colander, full of holes!

They then enter the bloodstream and bind our red blood cells together, causing clots that can lead to life-threatening embolisms. Besides lectins, other undigested protein molecules also make their way through the openings in this intestinal "sieve." Our sensitive immune system reacts immediately to this invasion but becomes disoriented as it tries to distinguish friend from foe. This happens because undigested protein molecules can resemble the molecules found on the outer layer of our cells. An autoimmune response thus occurs, which experts say is the cause of many illnesses.

But not all types of lectins are toxic. Precision Nutrition states,

> While many types of lectins cause negative reactions in the body, there are also health promoting lectins that can decrease the incidence of certain diseases. Furthermore, the body uses lectins to achieve many basic functions,

including cell to cell adherence, inflammatory modulation and programmed cell death.[190]

Avocados, for example, contain lectin but are considered a healthy food. Lectin foods can be made safe to eat through proper soaking and cooking, as well as fermenting and sprouting.

Saponins

Saponins, which appear in nearly all edible plants, are just as damaging. As plants, vegetables, and fruits mature, however, these chemicals practically disappear. In water, saponins produce foam just like soap does (hence their name—the Latin *sapo* means "soap"), which is why the parts of many saponin-rich plants are used as a soap substitute. They cause hemoglobin to enter the blood plasma because of the destruction of erythrocytes (hemolysis), whose main job is to transfer oxygen from the lungs to other tissues in the body. However, they are toxic when consumed in large amounts (e.g., in sweet chestnuts or unripe tomatoes). In low concentrations, they're basically harmless.

Cereal grains and legumes are the seeds of the parent plant and guarantee its natural development and reproduction. Evolution led them to develop certain characteristics to ensure these processes are carried out:

- They are resistant to digestion.
- They are excreted whole.

---

[190] Ryan Andrews, "All about Lectins," accessed May 1, 2018, https://www.precisionnutrition.com/all-about-lectins.

- They contain toxins that cannot be processed by the liver.
- Their hard covering protects the germ of the grain; not all living beings have teeth that can crush this covering.
- The simple and obvious question arises: With so many antinutrient components, are grains really fit for human consumption?

Homo essens: When and What?

From an evolutionary point of view, humans have learned to control such external threats as predators, low temperatures, the elements, and lack of food. But these enemies have been replaced by internal ones, which we ourselves introduce to our body by overusing medications, consuming harmful chemical "enhancers" and preservatives, and experiencing chronic stress.

Evolution clearly indicates that the human species has never consumed grains and sugar in such large amounts as we do today. This diet is a complete novelty to our body. Our biological drives are older than our intelligence by several million years. Food that quickly raises our blood sugar, or high glycemic food, is a recent addition to the diet of *Homo essens*.

Such food was only added to our diet around ten to twelve thousand years ago. Yet today, we eat so much of it that our delicate and sensitive endocrine system has been completely thrown out of balance. Our species' history shows that humans lived as hunters and gatherers, not farmers. Depending on where they traveled or were stopped by difficult conditions for a bit longer, early *Homo sapiens* got their food from a variety of wild, natural sources. These included various animals, birds, fruits, vegetables, nuts, seeds, and the green parts of many edible plants. Cereal grains like the ones we have today and sugar did not exist. Starting around ten thousand years ago, dramatic changes occurred in the human diet that now seem irreversible. Loren Cordain, author of the bestseller *The Paleo Diet*, notes,

> Cereal grains have fundamentally altered the foods to which our species had been originally adapted over eons of evolutionary experience. For better or for worse, we are no longer hunter-gatherers. However, our genetic makeup is still that of a Paleolithic hunter-gatherer, a species whose nutritional requirements are optimally adapted to wild meats, fruits, and vegetables, not to cereal grains. There is a significant body of evidence that suggests that cereal grains are less than optimal foods for humans and that the human genetic makeup and physiology may not be fully adapted to high levels of cereal grain consumption. We have wandered down a path toward absolute dependence upon cereal grains, a path for which there is no return.[191]

Admittedly, many archeological finds have given us examples of our cave-dwelling ancestors stocking various seeds

---

[191] Sisson, *The Primal Blueprint*, 15.

in their caverns, including wild grains. But animal products, especially meat and fats, remained the basis of their diet. The animals they hunted also provided fur, skin, and bones, which were used to make clothing, tools, and containers for water or food. As the Lakota people say, "We are all [humans, animals, insects, plants, minerals, and so on] related." Or as William Ralph Inge once wrote, "The whole of nature is a conjugation of the verb to eat, in the active and passive."[192]

Grains: Warnings and Recommendations

Many nutrition experts assure us that daily fiber consumption brings considerable benefits to our digestive tract. It also plays an important role in fighting colon cancer and may lower our blood cholesterol levels. Fiber appears exclusively in plant-based foods. So, you can find it in whole-grain products, fresh fruits, and vegetables. The highest amounts are found in wheat bran, peas, soy, corn bran, whole wheat bread, corn and oat flakes, rye bread, buckwheat groats, barley, and graham bread.

Dietitians say we should be eating thirty to forty grams of fiber each day. But should that come chiefly from grains? Like Francis Bacon, I believe, "Truth is the daughter of time, not of authority."

After thoroughly acquainting myself with these issues and after many years of personal experience and observation, I made the difficult decision to eliminate flour-based products from my diet. The longer I go without eating such products, the better I feel: my sense of well-being improves, I have more

---

[192] Pollan, *The Omnivore's Dilemma*, 6.

energy, I sleep deeper and better, my complexion is "brighter," and I have more positive thoughts and feel more open to new projects.

I feel so wonderful, in fact, that it would be a shame to throw it all away by giving in to a moment of personal weakness. I've come to realize that, when I break my resolutions, in just a few moments, I feel extremely tired, sleepy, and unable to concentrate. For now, I've no desire to treat myself to such mood swings and drains on my energy. Today, I look at baked goods, and what I see is not food. For me, they're just plastic props in store windows—decorations—and nothing more!

I've also observed something else: I can be quite creative in the kitchen! I'm always looking for new ways to spice up my menu, and I'm constantly discovering new, delicious, and healthy vegetables, fruits, and proteins that I hadn't known about before or that I had simply ignored the possibility of adding to my diet.

These novelties have given me so much creative inspiration, joy, and motivation to look onward. Of course, you start off with a bit of sacrifice, some difficulties, a few experiments, and a good dose of education, and then it's a matter of pure joy and delight for your palate and soul!

I recommend all my clients give up cereal grains for ninety days, followed by rolls, pasta, and other grains. The difference in their well-being and energy levels is so huge that—without exception—none of them ever wants to go back to flour-based delicacies.

In every discussion on grains, I regularly ask, "Have any of you ever tried avoiding baked goods for six weeks? Try it, and then we'll talk." I often add, "Observe your thoughts, emotions, and body as you do so!"

This experiment lets you free yourself from the prison of habit and bravely choose a new course. It's absolutely worth it! As the Greek sage Periander said, "Diligence is everything."

For those of you who don't know how, don't want to, or can't even imagine your life without grains, a healthier alternative would be to replace contemporary, cross-bred wheat and other seed monstrosities of civilization with such grains as

Spelt *(Triticum spelta)*

A variety of wheat, also known as dinkel wheat, spelt was still cultivated on a large scale in many regions of Europe at the beginning of the twentieth century, but wheat soon rose to dominate cereal farming. Spelt avoided destructive genetic modification, making it a grain that is truly ecologically pure and unchanged since ancient times and thus of great nutritional value. Spelt has more gluten than regular wheat, but you can easily remove it via fermentation. It also contains unsaturated fatty acids, which, in turn, contain phytosterols. An ancient grain, it is rich in vitamins A, E, D, B_1, and B_2, as well as niacin, phosphorus, iron, zinc, copper, manganese, and cobalt. Bread made from it has an intense, yeasty fragrance as well as a wonderful, singular taste. Spelt products retain their natural freshness for a long time. Saint Hildegard of Bingen, medieval nun and mystic, praised spelt in her writings on food and recipes (*Knowledge on Healing, Physica, and Scivias*): "The best grain is spelt. It is hot, rich and powerful. Eating it rectifies the flesh and provides healthy blood. It also creates a happy mind and puts joy in the human disposition."[193] This great twelfth-century mystic and healer believed spelt should be consumed in any form at least several times a day, as it had a positive effect on our blood, muscles, and psychological well-being. Later studies showed that its grains are very rich in silicic acid and zinc. The former has a significant impact on the condition of our hair, skin, and nails. It is essential for concentration and stimulating brain activity. Zinc, meanwhile, is an element that supports liver function and appears in many liver disease medications.

As an interesting aside, I'll just note that the entire spelt grain is used, even the separated chaff. Spelt hulls are used to make special, ecofriendly bedding, serving as filling for pillows, duvets, and mattresses. It is seen more and more often as a replacement for foam and other synthetic materials, as it promotes good sleep quality and joint regeneration while stopping excessive sweating.

Kamut (*Triticum turanicum*, Khorasan wheat)

The oldest wheat variety, this grain is surrounded by legend. The name *Kamut* has been trademarked by Kamut International Ltd. This grain's origins lie in ancient Egypt, and the name apparently signifies wheat in ancient hieroglyphics. Kamut grains were likely found in the pyramids, which is why it is also called "King Tut's wheat." It's difficult to say today how much of this is true and how much is just

---

[193] Saint Hildegard of Bingen, *Hildegard von Bingen's Physica*, trans. Priscilla Throop (Rochester: Inner Traditions / Bear & Co, 1998), 13.

sensational marketing by the Kamut Company meant to highlight its ancient character. After all, another story goes that the grain was carried on Noah's ark and was used as food for people, as well as animals during the great flood. Hence the grain's other name: "Prophet's wheat." "Camel's tooth" is yet another term for this grain, and though it may sound silly compared to the previous two, it is the most credible. This latter name is tied to the grain's size and shape. After all, it is much larger than normal wheat grains, with a distinctive curve and even a slight bump resembling a camel's hump. It is known by this name primarily in Turkey and neighboring countries. Kamut is very healthy, since it has also avoided biotechnological manipulation. It contains sodium, calcium, potassium, magnesium, sulfur, iron, and niacin, as well as the vitamins B_1, B_2, B_{12}, D, E, and K and large amounts of starch and protein.

Teff (lovegrass, annual bunch grass)

This is an ancient cereal grain that was first cultivated in northeast Africa centuries before our era. Teff is used mainly in baked goods, which are marked by their intense aroma and inimitable appearance. The tiny teff grains are ground and crushed whole, without removing the chaff. Bread made from teff is highly nutritious, since it boasts plenty of fiber, calcium, iron, and magnesium. Teff is also valued for its folic acid and antioxidant content. It's one of the few cereal grains known to humankind to contain *all* the amino acids and particularly high amounts of methionine, cysteine, and lysine.

Quinoa (*Chenopodium quinoa.*)

Quinoa is an annual plant that is not a true cereal but rather a member of the goosefoot (*Chenopodium*) family. Native to the Andes region in South America, quinoa has been cultivated for thousands of years (likely as many as five thousand) and is known as a staple of the Inca and Aztec diets. Interestingly, quinoa contains no gluten, so it can be consumed by those with celiac disease and does not cause damage to the body. Quinoa is beneficial to the digestive system and is a rich source of protein, numerous vitamins, and both macro- and microelements. It first caught Europeans' attention as an ancient and prized food in Peru, Ecuador, and Bolivia. As it turns out, quinoa contains 16 to 20 percent protein and high amounts of cysteine, lysine, and methionine, which are important amino acids for the human body. Quinoa is also prized for its high levels of iron, phosphorous, B vitamins, and healthy fats. However, because of the presence of antinutrients, the grain must be soaked before it is consumed.

Amaranth (*Amaranthus cruentus L.*)

Along with potatoes, corn, and beans, which have been cultivated for several thousand years, amaranth is one of the oldest staple crops of the Incas and Aztecs. Its nutritional value surpasses that of common wheat, and it now stands to become the grain of the twenty-first century. Like quinoa, amaranth does not contain gluten, does not cause digestive issues, and is not an allergen. It contains unsaturated fatty acids, which significantly limit the risk of heart disease and atherosclerosis. Amaranth reduces cholesterol levels, thus preventing circulatory diseases. It is rich in protein and squalene, an invaluable lipid that counteracts the aging process. Amaranth is not a typical cereal but in fact an annual member of the *Amaranthceae* family. It was long cultivated in Europe as food for pigs (hence the genus's unappetizing alternative name, pigweed). After all, the plant yields two or three crops per season. Animals that ate it were noted to be in excellent physical condition, did not get sick, and had high energy levels. Amaranth grains are also prized for their iron, calcium, magnesium, fiber, and vitamin D, A, E, and C content.

Buckwheat (*Fagopyrum esculentum.*)

An annual plant from the *Polygonaceae* family, originally from Mongolia, buckwheat produces thick, triangular "nuts" that turn amber-red when dried. It is cultivated for these exceptionally healthy and nutritious groats. Buckwheat contains calcium, vitamin E, and all the B vitamins. It is rich in essential amino acids, mainly lysine and arginine, which are not present in such large amounts in today's cereal grains. Buckwheat groats are gluten-free, so they are healthy and safe to consume for those with a gluten intolerance or celiac disease. However, they do contain phytic acid, which should be removed by soaking the buckwheat for several hours in salted water. But don't soak it for more than seven hours, since it forms an unappetizing mush when left to sit longer. Buckwheat groats are relatively rich in phytase, a useful enzyme that breaks down phytic acid. This is enormously beneficial for us. I highly recommend buckwheat and give it my wholehearted stamp of approval!

Oats (*Avena sativa.*)

I've noticed that many people have an extremely emotional attitude toward oatmeal—that is, oat flakes boiled in milk. They can't imagine starting their day without their oatmeal. Sometimes, they even serve this traditional dish to their children, completely confident that they're doing something good for them. What is it about oatmeal that makes it so popular? Samuel Johnson, the English writer and lexicographer, defined oats as "a grain, which in England is generally given to horses, but in Scotland appears to support the people."[194] It was first discovered as a weed growing wild in barley fields in Russia, North Africa, and the Middle East. Yet, inhabitants of the cooler climates of Scotland, Ireland, and England quickly began to cultivate it. It was first sown in Massachusetts fields around 1600 CE, which is how it landed on American consumers' tables as the popular oatmeal. The grains used to make oatmeal are rich in B vitamins, calcium, iron, phosphorus, and potassium. They contain healthier fats than other grains. Oats are low in gluten but high in phytic acid. Therefore, it's extremely important—even necessary—to give your oats a long soak in salted water before making your favorite oatmeal.[195]

---

[194] Samuel Johnson, "Dictionary of the English Language," accessed March 22, 2017, http://www.bl.uk/learning/langlit/dic/johnson/oats/oats.html.
[195] The recipe is in the appendix.

Remember, phytic acid deprives our bodies of minerals, particularly calcium and magnesium. While it's true that oatmeal boasts many nutrients, that means very little if the human corpus doesn't absorb them and on top of it all is forced to use up its reserves in the process! Phytic acid is present in the bran of the oat grain and may have detoxifying properties. So, it provides certain health benefits at first, only to cause vitamin deficiencies, allergies, and intestinal issues later. This happens especially when the grains are not properly prepared for consumption.

Millet (*Panicum miliaceum L.*)

Millet is a grass species that is widely cultivated in tropical areas, as well as some countries in more temperate climes. In addition to sorghum, it is the primary staple grain for millions, especially in poorer regions. Millet has been cultivated in areas such as India, Central Africa, Myanmar, Thailand, China, and parts of Russia since time immemorial. It was brought to Europe in the Middle Ages, several centuries before potatoes and corn. Millet was cultivated mainly for its edible groats and was also used as poultry feed. It does not contain gluten and has a low phytic acid content. In addition to protein, the B vitamins, vitamins E and C, and niacin, millet is also rich in silicon, an essential nutrient for maintaining flexible bones during the natural aging process. Unfortunately, millet's structure also contains a substance known as goitrogen, which hinders thyroid function. People with thyroid problems should exclude it from their diet.

As an interesting aside, the ancient Slavs cultivated a variety of millet known in Polish as "bloody finger" millet (although English seems to prefer names like "crabgrass" or "hairy finger grass") because of its slender green or ruddy leaves, which were used in a wide range of culinary applications. Today, it is treated like a weed.

Who knows? Perhaps scientists will one day place it back on its former pedestal, and this variety will enjoy its own agricultural renaissance. After all, this has already happened to all the ancient grains that science has brought back, setting off a certain vogue for them. This includes most of those that I've presented here. I'm curious to see what properties this mysterious millet of my Slavic ancestors is hiding, just waiting to be discovered by contemporary consumers.

Rice (*Oryza sativa*)

Rice is an annual species of the grass family cultivated over all of Southeast Asia in tropical and subtropical climates, as well as in North America and in the western parts of the Gulf Coastal Plain and some regions of Mexico. It is the primary staple food for most people in East Asia. The Japanese and Chinese consume over 45 kilograms (99 pounds) of rice per person per year. Rice requires a warm climate and very moist soil, and artificially irrigated fields can sometimes yield two or three harvests a year. Macrobiotic enthusiasts consider it to be the ideal grain, in which the energy of yin and yang are in perfect balance. People of the West, however, shouldn't hurry to adopt Asia's rice tradition completely and uncritically, since they aren't adapted to it the way native consumers are. East Asians tend to have a larger pancreas and salivary glands, making them ideally suited to a diet full of rice dishes. Westerners who want to follow this dietary model, meanwhile, may suffer serious health consequences. Rice grains do not contain gluten and are relatively low in phytic acid. Brown rice is high in phytates and has more B vitamins, iron, vitamin E, and protein than other types of rice. Soaking brown rice will not effectively eliminate phytates because brown rice lacks the enzyme phytase; it thus requires a starter.[196]

So-called wild rice is also a good, healthy alternative to other grains. It contains many amino acids and B vitamins. Wild rice is rich in magnesium, potassium, phosphorus, and zinc, yet low in fat, which is why it is best to eat it with plenty of butter or olive oil cooled in the broth. Rice is consumed in a variety of forms, including rice porridge, rice flour, puffed rice, and rice noodles. It is the second most-cultivated grain in the world after wheat. Rice has more starch than any other grain and should be soaked for at least eight hours in hot water with a little fresh whey, lemon juice, or vinegar and then cooked in broth and butter. Thanks to the two or three crops it yields each year, rice has been and still is a symbol of fertility, good fortune, and sustenance. To this day, people in many cultures throw it over the heads of newlyweds so that fate will favor them and bring them many healthy children. This magical, symbolic gesture underscores the significance of this grain in human life.

---

[196] Ramiel Nagel, "Living with Phytic Acid," The Weston A. Price Foundation, last updated March 26, 2010, https://www.westonaprice.org/health-topics/vegetarianism-and-plant-foods/living-with-phytic-acid/.

A Few Words about Nuts and Seeds

In its article "Living with Phytic Acid," the WAPF (Weston A. Price Foundation) states that not enough thorough, responsible research has been done to develop an effective and simple method for removing phytic acid from nuts and seeds. We do know that soaking nuts and seeds in salted water for several hours and then drying them at an appropriate temperature gives us a crunchy delight that is easily digested and does not cause intestinal discomfort.

Nuts are full of healthy fats and boast many wonderful health properties. However, you can't just eat as many as you want. A single handful of nuts is an appropriate, sufficient amount.

Walnut and hazel trees were prized in the past for their seeds' undeniable merits. In ancient Ireland, hazel was a sacred tree; willfully cutting one down was a crime punishable by death. It was a magical tree whose fruit could last for a long time and guarantee relief from hunger. Dowsers used hazel branches to detect underground water sources, while magicians and diviners foretold the future and drove off thunderbolts and evil spirits with them.

Hazelnuts, which often appear in twos and threes on hazel branches, became a symbol of nature's vital force and fertility. They were eagerly given to loved ones and friends on solemn feast days. This tradition continues to this day at Christmas and New Year's as an expression of friendship and love.

Grains, nuts, and seeds have been known to humankind for ages. In many cultures, they are prized for their nutritional value, which is what led to their cultivation in the first place.

We can find descriptions not only in the Bible but also in the oldest jottings of ancient civilizations.

Today, it has become something of a trend to return to those grains that have been cultivated since the most ancient times and attempt to preserve their original form and genetic structure. Hence the belief (confirmed by numerous studies) in their greater, undeniable value has brought about today's veritable renaissance of ancient crops and their recipes.

Remember

- From an evolutionary perspective, humankind has never consumed grains or sugars in such large amounts.
- High-glycemic foods are an unnatural and unhealthy presence in our diet.
- Attempting to eliminate flour-based foods from our diet may bring about an amazing and healthy renewal of our bodies and their functioning.
- Removing phytic acid from the grains we eat is an absolute necessity; this is done by soaking them in salted water for several hours.
- The fiber, amino acids, and antioxidants that are so vital for our bodies can be obtained from sources other than whole-grain food.
- We should pay close attention to the grains, seeds, and nuts we consume, even in highly sophisticated dishes, so that they don't end up dominating our diet.

CHAPTER 13

A MEETING WITH LIFE-GIVING CHEMICALS OR VITAMINS

> During the past two decades, a steady stream of
> high-quality studies evaluating dietary supplements
> has yielded predominantly disappointing results
> about potential health benefits, whereas evidence
> of harm has continued to accumulate.[197]
> —Pieter A. Cohen in *JAMA*

The National Institutes of Health has spent more than $2.4 billion studying synthetic vitamins and minerals, only to find out they really don't work.[198] Vitamins and minerals *cannot* and *should not* be consumed in the form of isolated concentrates and pills.

But before we start our discussion about the effectiveness of synthetic supplements or the lack thereof, I would like

---

[197] Piter A. Cohen, "The Supplement Paradox Negligible Benefits, Robust Consumption," accessed May 22, 2018, https://jamanetwork.com/journals/jama/article-abstract/2565733?redirect=true via http://bigthink.com/21st-century-spirituality/24-billion-later-vitamins-and-supplements-appear-to-have-no-value.

[198] Derek Beres, "Multivitamins Are Not Only Ineffective, But Dangerous," accessed May 23, 2018, http://bigthink.com/21st-century-spirituality/24-billion-later-vitamins-and-supplements-appear-to-have-no-value.

to begin this chapter with a story I heard my aunt tell as I lounged in her garden, munching on fresh cherries.

In 2005, I met up with an old school friend who had lived in Chicago for years. Poland's complicated history had severed my friend's ties with family and friends, violently uprooting her and forcing her into emigration as an "alien being," who would go about discovering the new world around her with an anxious child's wonder.

She told me about the astonishment that bombarded her day in and day out in seemingly trivial situations. Orange juice that didn't come from oranges; milk that wouldn't sour for weeks; ripe, healthy-looking yet tasteless strawberries; large, smooth, shiny apples packed in colorful tissue paper that "you'd be better off not buying or eating"—all of this became part of her American reality.

Her new American friends tried to guide her through this world, but when it came to food, her unease and caution grew. She decided she would protect herself with artificial vitamin, protein, and mineral supplements, while limiting her diet only to the food products she trusted, which were few.

This did not go well for her. She felt tired, distracted, weak, lacking in energy, never well-rested. After having some tests done, it turned out that, despite her resolutions, she was deficient in some basic nutrients, since she wasn't eating *fresh* fruits, vegetables, healthy fats or fresh meat every day.

As my friend told me this story, she was happily swinging on my garden swing and then, reaching out both her hands, grabbed some cherries straight from the tree and ate them with relish. I looked around at my garden. Moved and full of pride, I realized how each morning I could walk out in my pajamas and enjoy fragrant, wild strawberries, currants of three different colors, gooseberries, peaches, apples, and nuts straight from the bush or tree, confident they were the healthy products of my husband's and my collaboration with *nature*, which had granted us its unbelievable wealth.

Well, I took with me to Amsterdam some little jars, full of fragrant, appetizing preserves that my daughter had made herself for the first time in her life at my host's side. When I gave them to some close friends, they greeted my offerings with delight and great culinary interest.

I don't mean to suggest that you go out and start up an organic garden and become self-sufficient like some medieval monk. I'd only prefer you put a special effort into finding healthy food that is obviously rich in nutrients and that will ensure your body's natural balance.

We should take great care to avoid the situation recounted in this particular Old-World message: well into old age (more than one hundred years old), the popular and respected ancient Greek orator Gorgias was asked whether it'd be easy for him to leave this world when his time came. "Yes, very easy," he replied. "It would be as if I were happily leaving a dilapidated, rotting house."[199]

With a proper diet and lifestyle, we can maintain good mental and physical fitness for years without letting our bodies fall into ruin or extreme disrepair.

Today, it is difficult to say exactly when and in what conditions our ancestors first noticed that certain foods were worth eating because they guaranteed well-being, sharp eyesight, good health, strong bones, and hard teeth. Yet somehow, thanks to their intuition and experience, they did.

Research into the lifestyles of many ancient societies in various regions of the world shows that small-scale agriculture appeared very early near human dwellings, while later ages even left behind literature on the subject. One example is Virgil, the Roman poet from the first century BCE, in his work *Georgics*. This is a didactic poem in four books, dedicated to farming, arboriculture, viniculture, livestock farming, and beekeeping (apiculture), and it draws the reader in with its great love and respect for nature.

---

[199] Author's own translation from the Polish.

The work includes the beautiful and colorful short tale of a certain old man from Corycus, who unexpectedly came into possession of a bit of wasteland that was unfit for plowing, planting a vineyard, or even grazing sheep. As the verse goes, "planting cabbages here and there among the brambles, and white lilies and vervain and fine-seeded poppies, in happiness he equaled the wealth of kings, and returning home late at night he used to load his table with an unbought banquet."[200]

In those times, some plant species were already considered to have "strength-giving material." Medieval scholar-monks also used this observation. Their monasteries were typically surrounded by gardens, where, throughout the centuries, they patiently and diligently cultivated vegetables, medicinal and culinary herbs, and fruit trees and bushes, as well as flowers to decorate holy images and altars. Such experiences were recorded along with scientific commentary by gardening pioneer and Archbishop of Cologne Albertus Magnus (St. Albert the Great) in his work *De vegetabilibus*.

We can thank these monastic communities living in harmony with Mother Nature for numerous insights into the beneficial effects of many plant species consumed by humans. As St. Hildegard of Bingen, founder of natural and herbal medicine, as well as ecology, described their properties, "In each of God's creatures His wonderful works are thus hidden: in animals and fish, birds, in herbs and flowers and trees." The rules for living developed by this Benedictine scholar are still relevant and seemingly universal. According

200   Virgil, *Georgics*, trans. by H. R. Fairclough, accessed March 22, 2017, http://www.theoi.com/Text/VirgilGeorgics2.html#4.

to Hildegard,[201] to be healthy and satisfied with life, you should do the following:

- draw your vital energy from the four elements of the world
- eat and drink right
- find the right rhythm of movement and calm, and thus work and rest
- understand sleep and waking as counterbalancing forces
- "eliminate bad humors" and "fortify" good ones

In medieval Central and Eastern Europe, valuable foods included peas, fava beans, dried and pickled mushrooms, fresh cucumbers and pickles, carrots, fresh and sour cabbage, turnips, garlic, and onions. Orchards were home to apples, sour and sweet cherries, plums, and pears.

In Mediterranean countries, this fruit and vegetable assortment also included local crops typical for the region and climate. Many exotic spices were also brought from the most distant corners of the Far East and traded in the markets of the largest European cities. In the tenth century, the leading city in this respect was Mogontiacum (today's Mainz), the undisputed center of the spice trade, supplying seasonings to inhabitants across Northern and Eastern Europe.

However, the situation radically changed following Columbus's discoveries. Farming expanded to include new plants, exotic dishes appeared on tables, and greenhouses

---

[201] Hildegard of Bingen, *Sensacje i porady na każdy dzień* [Sensations and advice for every day], 13.

and hothouses sprouted up in gardens in which heretofore unknown fruits, vegetables, and flowers from far-off lands grew. From that time on, gardeners, orchard keepers, and farmers had unlimited access to an extraordinary diversity of biological material, as well as valuable natural and agricultural resources.

All of this contributed significantly to an improvement in Europeans' overall health, and they were no longer decimated by such severe epidemics as the Black Death, which spread in the fourteenth century. With a nutrient-rich diet, they developed greater immunity to many illnesses, which their stronger, better-nourished bodies were able to resist. Note that here we're talking about "strength-giving materials," "fortifying good humors," "miraculous works," and not *vitamins*. That term would appear quite a bit later.

In the mid-nineteenth century, the German chemist Justus von Liebig noted that the only things necessary for human and animal life are sugars, protein, fats, salts, and water. Yet, as early as 1905, the Dutch professor Cornelius Adrianus Pekelharing observed that milk contained an "unknown substance" of great nutritional significance. In 1912, the Polish biochemist Casimir Funk coined the term *vitamine* (from the Latin *vitalis*, meaning life-giving, capable of life; *vita* "life"; *aminum* "amine") for a chemical compound he discovered in food that proved necessary for life. He isolated this substance from the husk of rice grains and noticed that it prevented the disease beriberi.

Interestingly, when this discovery was first reported in the medical literature in Poland, the original term was translated literally as *życian* (from Polish *życie*, or life), which clearly emphasized its vital significance.

Today, science recognizes around thirty chemical elements as forming the basic building blocks of living organisms. They appear either as ions or chemical compounds. These include macro-elements—those found in larger amounts (calcium, phosphorus, magnesium, sodium, and potassium)—and micro-elements, or trace elements, which are present in smaller amounts (iron, selenium, fluorine, chromium, cobalt, iodine, vanadium, nickel, arsenic, manganese, molybdenum, copper, and zinc).

In addition to these elements, vitamins also play a key role. Without them, the processes that keep us alive cannot be performed properly. This can manifest itself in various ways, from symptoms of a disordered metabolism to scurvy, blindness, beriberi, and eventually death.

Vitamins are organic microelements that are necessary for the normal metabolic process to take place in the human body. They are not processed by the body into energy in the way fats, proteins, and sugars are. Most are not produced by the human body and thus must be provided via food.

Each of these naturally occurring organic compounds fulfils a specific, crucial function and is not only desirable but ultimately essential to the functioning and development of our organs, tissues, and cells. These parts of the human body can fight off illnesses, stay healthy, and prolong our lives, all thanks to vitamins. The entire gamut of known vitamins is divided into two groups: fat-soluble and water-soluble.

The first group includes vitamins A, D, E, and K, while vitamin C and the B vitamins belong to the latter. Fat-soluble vitamins can be stored by the body and thus do not need to be supplied daily. Vitamin D, for example, can be stored for three to five months. It should be added that an excess of each of these vitamins is not excreted in the urine, and too much of them can be toxic. Water-soluble vitamins can be taken in larger doses. Vitamin C and the B vitamins (except B_{12}) are not stored by the body and should be consumed regularly.

In-depth knowledge about vitamins and their role in human life is relatively recent, but people have long noted from experience and observation that certain herbs, fruits, and vegetables must contain some invisible, valuable substances that give us life and can return us to strength and health. Hence, they made extraordinary efforts to have such a natural pharmacy nearby in their home gardens.

In Ancient Egypt and Greece, eating carrots was recommended for so-called night blindness (nyctalopia). Today, we know that this impairment (poor vision at dusk and at night) is caused by a deficiency in vitamin A, which is found in foods like carrots.

Many different factors undoubtedly contributed to humankind's ancient awareness of the significant relationship between food from nature and our health. This knowledge was sometimes closely guarded by physicians, healers, priests, and monks. However, such actions proved unable to quench human curiosity and our determination to know these secrets and alleviate our health problems.

Today, it doesn't matter whether this happened because of our ancestors' intuition, common sense, or dogged persistence. What's important is that they *understood* very early on the vital power that is contained in the invisible substances found in natural foods. Their powers of observation and desire to help themselves and others worked without fail for centuries, eventually paying off in our modern era of extensive research on vitamins.

A milestone in this field was achieved by James Lind, a Scottish physician and pioneer of naval hygiene in the Royal Navy. He observed that scurvy decimated European sailors in particular, and reliable sources backed this up. In 1499, Vasco da Gama lost 116 members of his 170-person crew, while Magellan lost 208 of 230 sailors in 1520. Scurvy was the primary culprit behind these enormous losses. After observing the crews of ships from the East, Admiral Sir Richard Hawkins recommended drinking lemon and orange juice. This custom was quickly given up, however, and Hawkins's observations were largely ignored.

During George Anson's famed 1740–1742 voyage, the first ten months saw the loss of 1,400 out of 1,900 men. Most were reported to have contracted scurvy. Between 1500 and 1800, scurvy caused the deaths of at least two million sailors. According to James Lind, scurvy led to more deaths in the British fleet than battles with the French or Spanish.

In 1753, he published his famous *Treatise of the Scurvy*, in which he demonstrates that citrus fruit juice prevents the disease and, even once the disease has appeared, quickly reverses its damage and life-threatening symptoms. The results of his studies provoked debate among English physicians, who couldn't come to a consensus, and Lind's discoveries were ignored for the next forty years. One hundred-thousand British sailors paid for this delay with their lives.

Scurvy is caused by a vitamin C deficiency, but in Lind's time, the very concept of vitamins, much less the substance itself, was unknown. This tragedy was completely preventable. All they needed to do was to drink water with fresh lemon juice daily or follow the example of James Cook, who—paying no heed to the experts' feuding—on his first long voyage (1768–1771) took orange and lemon syrup, sauerkraut, and wort, an intermediate product in the beer- and mead-brewing process. Thus, he had a nearly complete set of vitamins on board in the form of natural foods.

It should be added that similar treatments had existed in many cultures since prehistoric times and were passed down from generation to generation. For example, trans-Atlantic travelers who reached North America in 1536, exhausted by the voyage and scurvy, camped at the mouth of the St. Lawrence River and were saved from certain death by white pine needle tea brewed regularly by the natives. Later studies revealed that 100 grams of this brew contains as much as 50 grams of vitamin C.

The therapeutic effects of fresh meat were well-known among whalers and those who studied the Arctic and Inuit, who used such meat to give strength to the weary at sea. It turns out that everything in life is much simpler than it seems. There are those, however, who are only superficially interested in the world around them yet truly care about nothing, and it is they who tend to jump to rash conclusions and disregard ancient, tried-and-true solutions.

James Lind was certainly not one of them; he also observed how distilling seawater could produce fresh water. The researcher's perseverance paid off, and he was recognized as a pioneer of preventative medicine who stressed the remarkable role that a proper diet played in human health and life.

In 1905, the English physician William Fletcher noted that a vitamin B_1 deficiency caused the illness beriberi, a severe form of avitaminosis (or rather, hypovitaminosis). In those days, the disease appeared primarily among Asian populations. The scientist observed that only those who ate white polished rice were affected. Patients who received brown, unpolished rice, which contained vitamin B in its husks, recovered. This experiment included 123 patients and eventually led to the discovery of thiamine—vitamin B_1—and other B vitamins.

The Polish biochemist Casimir Funk, mentioned previously, continued his predecessor's research in 1912. He discovered the presence of vitamin B_1 in rice husks and other foods, including yeast, milk, and beef brain. The scientist also coined the term *vitamine*. It should be added that its first half, *vita*, was accepted without any reservations, but the second—*amine*—suggested that the nitrogen compounds (or amines) present in thiamine were common to all vitamins; this observation was later refuted, and the -*e* was dropped.

Today, the full chemical names of these substances are being used more and more often in lieu of the term *vitamin* plus a letter, and now we see the traditional vitamin nomenclature only in popular literature, advice books, and advertising. Casimir Funk was the first to predict that a deficiency in some vitamins could cause many illnesses, such as rickets, scurvy, and pellagra. He was convinced that these substances have an enormous impact on vitality, health, and the quality and length of human life.

In 1930, a veritable avalanche of scientific discoveries led to the determination of the biochemical functions of different vitamins and the cataloguing of their influences and effects on the human body. Articles began to be published on a mass scale, appearing not only in scientific publications but also in popular magazines and newspapers. Society was eager to learn about vitamins and consciously introduced them into their daily lives, thus signaling that health is an important individual and public issue.

This attitude is illustrated perfectly by Brian R. Clement's words:

> We must start with a simple biological fact of life: Vitamins and minerals are essential to human health, and the human body is unable to manufacture most of what it needs. These nutrients must be obtained from the food that we eat and the supplements we take derived from food.[202]

Research on vitamins continues, and food as a scientific subject has turned out to be more mysterious and complicated than scientists first imagined. Food triggers an unbelievable number of processes and chemical relationships, which together form a highly sensitive and delicate structure of moderation and harmony. Its disruption by even the tiniest wrong component not only leads to shock and chaos for the human corpus but, most important, threatens our

---

[202] Clement, *Supplements Exposed*, 24.

psychological and physical health. Consuming the right food thus becomes a source of life, strength, and health.

Vitamins and microelements are biocatalysts that play a key role in the body's biological processes. In the small amounts found in the food we consume, they deliver tangible, positive effects to each of the living cells in our bodies, restoring harmony and internal order to its functioning. They cause a natural surge in strength, energy, health, and youth.

The pioneering researchers of these mysterious substances made an enormous contribution to deciphering individual vitamins' structure and determining their role in our health. The watershed moment came once these compounds could be isolated and synthesized, thus allowing preparations to be made that were packed with more beneficial elements than natural food.

This led to the mistaken conclusion that vitamins and minerals can and should be consumed in the form of isolated concentrates and pills that supplement our daily diet. In the wake of these conclusions, industries, sensing great business opportunities, grew up and soon launched aggressive advertising campaigns promoting technologically produced "healthy additives."

These days, scientists know that vitamins do not exist as individual forms working in isolation but are complex compounds that form part of a living, biological whole. This is an extraordinary "collective structure," formed in nature to fulfill specific functions.

All vitamins give their optimal results in the presence of naturally occurring cooperators and accompanying factors, such as trace elements, enzymes, coenzymes, and other vitamins, tocopherols, and phytonutrients, whose roles in our bodies are still the subject of extensive scientific research. This extraordinary natural interaction and its mechanisms cannot be recreated in laboratory conditions, making it impossible to introduce them to living organisms in an identical form through dietary supplements that would work as they are naturally programmed to.

There are four elements of natural foods, created by the power of nature (and not humankind), that have not yet been sufficiently analyzed by most chemists. These are hormones, oxygen content, phytochemical levels (plant-based chemical compounds), and enzymes (protein substances that catalyze the metabolic processes of living organisms), of which several thousand have already been discovered and with no end in sight.

All these elements support and stimulate the work of vitamins and minerals. Without their participation and help, vitamins and minerals are worthless. Each of these components is a factor of utmost importance, together fulfilling all the body's nutritional requirements and electromagnetic needs, and each is of fundamental significance to our cellular health and functioning.

Vitamin C

Let's start by taking a closer look at the most popular vitamin—vitamin C—as an illustration of these points. Among its many roles, vitamin C, also known as ascorbic acid, plays an important part in processes such as tissue growth and repair, capillary wall integrity, lactation, and proper adrenal function. It also contributes significantly to the production of collagen, a structural protein in the human body. This vitamin speeds up wound healing and is a strong antioxidant. It is most effective when found in natural food products that contain minerals, rutin, and other analogues.

Vitamin C works in synergy with vitamin E. Large amounts of isolated ascorbic acid lead to disruptions to the body's natural balance and deficiencies in vitamin P bioflavonoids, which strengthen our absorption of vitamin C. Smokers, drinkers, hypoglycemic people, and those who eat large amounts of meat have a greater need for vitamin C.

The vitamin is found in many fruits and vegetables, as well as in some animal organs. Many foods known as *superfoods* are rich in vitamin C, e.g., camu camu, acerola (the fruit of this shrub is one of the vitamin's richest sources), rose hips, bee pollen, raw cocoa, unpasteurized milk, quince, and white pine needles. Vitamin C aids iron absorption. Women taking birth control, as well as residents of industrial areas and large cities, need more of it. Smog containing carbon monoxide and heavy metals damages the vitamin. Birth control pills can deplete your body of several B vitamins (riboflavin, B6, B12, and folic acid), vitamin C, magnesium, and zinc.[203]People who are deficient in copper should not consume vitamin C, because vitamin C lowers copper levels, which can seriously compromise the immune system.

---

[203] Monica Reinagel, "How Birth Control Pills Affect Your Nutritional Needs," accessed July 20, 2018, https://www.scientificamerican.com/article/how-birth-control-pills-affect-your-nutritional-needs/.

Vitamin P

Vitamin P is a collective term for bioflavonoids. It stimulates bile production, lowers cholesterol, helps regulate menstruation, has antibacterial properties, and helps prevent cataracts. It works with vitamin C to protect and repair capillary and artery walls and thins the blood, lowering its coagulability. In nature, these vitamins always appear together, inseparable like conjoined twins!

One place where they can be found together is albedo—the white substance beneath the peel of citrus fruits—in which citrin is the form of vitamin P that contributes to vitamin C absorption. This is a well-coordinated, hardworking team that is responsible for cancer resistance. It also prevents respiratory diseases, restores male fertility, fights periodontal disease, and, most important, slows down our biological clock by increasing white blood cell counts in folks over fifty.

So, if you take chemically produced (synthetic) isolated vitamin C, its only effect is to empty your wallet! Interestingly enough, no matter what manufacturer information you find on the package insert, 90 percent of vitamin C is a synthetic product produced in Chinese factories.

Vitamin B

As many as seventeen water-soluble vitamins are labelled with the letter B, often with an additional number. They exist in various proportions in many food products, but all of them work in synergy, supporting or stimulating each other's individual tasks. Each of these vitamins is helpless without the others.

They should appear in our daily diet, since they are not stored in our bodies. The B vitamins influence the condition of our nervous system, our intellectual ability, and energy release from carbohydrates. They help maintain healthy hair, skin, and nails, and they work together to produce hydrochloric acid and help us absorb magnesium.

The B vitamins participate in too many processes to list them all here, and numerous research centers around the world continue to track and study them. The important conclusion here is that taking a synthetic "B complex" configuration, which most often contains six B vitamins (sometimes also with vitamin B_{12} and folic acid, vitamin M), does not guarantee a full set of B vitamins, the natural proportions between them, or their individual activity in the processes assigned to them by biology.

Vitamin D

Vitamin D may have twelve components, each of which contributes in its own way to bone and teeth development and to calcium and phosphorus absorption. Vitamin A plays a similar role in these processes. Calcium absorption is not possible without vitamin D, magnesium, and fat. Moreover, calcium and phosphorus must work in tandem in a proper ratio to one another and in the presence of sufficient vitamin D— factors that may be disrupted by the improper composition of synthetic preparations. As you can see, buying calcium or magnesium by itself makes no sense whatsoever.

This extensive, seemingly unfinished list of important factors in our health and lives has prompted dieticians and doctors to recognize that efforts to provide them in the form of synthetic supplements are insufficient and even futile. Of course, they admit that isolated, synthetic vitamins that are administered immediately and prescribed over the long term bring positive results and can save human health and lives in the case of certain health conditions, incidents, and accidents.

These extreme medical situations aside, the only optimal source of vitamins our bodies can assimilate comes from wholesome, unprocessed, natural, fresh food. Getting nutrients from the source—from your diet—ensures the proper functioning of the body and a high quality of life.

What a lot of people don't realize is that supplement use, particularly when taking supplements in large doses, may increase your risk for disease. Not only are supplements no substitute for whole foods, they could pose a health risk—studies point to a link between heavy supplementation and an increased risk for heart disease and cancer. For example, a 2006 study involving 170,000 people found that supplementing with high doses of vitamins A, C, E, and beta-carotene may increase the risk of developing intestinal cancer. Other studies have found a link between large doses of vitamin E and a greater risk for both cancer and heart disease. And a 2005 John Hopkins study revealed that taking megavitamins can increase the risk for an early death—which is pretty startling considering people are taking supplements to *increase* health and vitality.[204]

---

[204] Paul Offit, "Pandora's Lab: Seven Stories of Science Gone Wrong," *National Geographic*, Washington 2016, via http://bigthink.com/21st-century-spirituality/24-billion-later-vitamins-and-supplements-appear-to-have-no-value.

No chemically produced substance with a label slapped on it reading "natural" or "identical to nature" can replace a properly prepared meal made from at least 55 percent raw ingredients! Nothing can justify eating meals that have been stripped of their natural nutrients and then popping a handful of colorful pills! That's no way to get strength, energy, or vitality. Paul Chek described it very well in one of his books: "Vitamins are like nails, and your macronutrients are like the wood used to build a boat. It doesn't matter if you use golden nails, building a boat out of junk wood will only result in a useless boat that sinks, taking your golden nails right to the bottom."[205]

Nothing proper, sound, or long-lasting can be built from materials of dubious quality. In the case of vitamins and minerals, this depends on the class and type of soil and the farming methods used. Nitrogen fertilizers initially provided high yields in large part due to intensive use of the minerals contained in the soil. With time, this led to soil depletion, and the quality of the food obtained from it fell dramatically. "Rowing harder doesn't help if the boat is headed in the wrong direction"—this reflection by Kenichi Ohmae perfectly sums up these absurd actions.

Some theories say the discovery of agriculture represented humans' first fall from the state of nature; in that case, the discovery of synthetic fertilizers is surely the second. In 1909, Fritz Haber—a Jewish chemist whose work led to Zyklon B, the gas used in Nazi concentration camps—found a simple way to synthesize ammonia for fertilizer from nitrogen and

---

[205] Chek, *How to Eat, Move and Be Healthy*, 47.

hydrogen. In 1920, he won the Nobel Prize for "improving the standards of agriculture and the well-being of mankind." However, what really happened is, in Michael Pollan's words, "[I]nstead of eating exclusively from the sun, humanity now began to sip petroleum."[206] Over the past fifty years, the vitamin and mineral content in fruit and vegetables from large commercial plantations has fallen drastically. Fertile soil should contain fifty-five minerals to feed the plants growing in it. Unfortunately, such soil is so wastefully exploited that it now contains only two![207] These figures speak for themselves.

In the name of profit and in highly sophisticated ways, humankind can cause thoughtless, utter destruction of the environment on which our lives depend. Without any resistance, human beings exploit all the elements of their own ecological community, without thinking about the consequences of their actions, and build on its ruins a synthetic world "identical to nature." A person could even call this unimaginative, irresponsible, and cynical policy the brutal rape of nature.

Primitive cultures treated the nature surrounding them with respect and humility, realizing their dependence on it. It may seem strange to a Westerner that Tagalogs in the Philippines, before picking a flower or cutting down a tree, ask the spirits of these plants for their permission and forgiveness.

Interfering in nature's harmony and laws and damaging the environment violates a taboo and threatens their existence.

---

[206] Pollan, *The Omnivore's Dilemma*, 45.
[207] J. Colquhoun and C. Ledesma, *Food Matters* (Australia: Permacology Productions, 2008), DVD, interview with Charlotte Gerson.

Conscientious food consumers and most especially producers should reflect on the attitudes presented here.

Fertile soil that is rich in numerous minerals (including trace elements) forms the *foundation of health* for every form of life on our planet. While research in this area is far from complete, we do know the factors that determine the nutritional content of fruits and vegetables are numerous. This means we can impact the nutritional density of our food. Genetic modification, the quality of the soil we plant our seeds in, and how much the plants are subjected to disease or pests all impact the final outcome. Even the after-harvest period plays a role in how many nutrients are in your fruits and veggies—the time from harvest to consumption as well as the storage and transportation methods involved factor into the nutrition equation.

The oxidation process is the main reason for the loss of vitamins from food, which is why fruit and vegetable juices should be consumed immediately after being made—in a few minutes, they become nothing more than sugar water. The same is true for salads and desserts. All their ingredients should be sliced just before serving, so that as many of their nutrients are preserved as possible.

Fruits and vegetables should be eaten while still quite fresh, ideally right after being picked from the tree or bush or just as they're dug up from the soil. The longer they're transported, stored, processed, and preserved, the fewer nutrients they have. This means where you choose to purchase your produce from will impact how many vitamins, minerals, antioxidants, and other nutrients you'll get from your food.

This is why we should do our shopping at local farmers' markets and consume in-season food from our own local region.

Purchasing any exotic food items that have undergone a long journey and have been sprayed with preservatives and rinsed with antifungal and antispoilage agents makes no sense! The importance of well-thought-out purchases may be illustrated by the wise and firm warning known even to the ancient Israelites: "A scholar is not allowed to live in a city without vegetables."

In Elizabethan England, most of the streets of London had names signaling where one could easily buy fresh foods. There were Bread Street, Milk Street, and Fish Street Hill, whose shops and stalls offered daily displays of goods that would find their way straight from the supplier into customers' hands, with no need to search or wait in line. There were also innumerable small marketplaces just outside the city, where stallholders would sell poultry, dairy, vegetables, fruit, and flowers bought from neighboring villagers.

This is still the case in many regions of the world today. You just need to find these places and begin to value them more than the monolithic supermarkets. And once we've found, selected, and purchased this food and brought it home, we should remember that some vitamins are completely or partially damaged in the cooking process, while others go untouched and may even have a stronger effect. This is true for such foods as tomatoes, cabbage, and slow-cooked bone broths, for example.

Traditional techniques for fermenting vegetables enrich them with vitamins, minerals, and beneficial bacterial cultures. In many cultures, barrels of sauerkraut, pickles, and pickled mushrooms became a primary source of these natural riches. Germany, Poland, and Russia have preserved this tradition to the present, while in Balkan and Caucasian cuisine, other regional vegetables, such as peppers, are also pickled.

A great variety of spices are used in pickling, making these foods not only vitamin-rich but also true delicacies that are the pride of every thoughtful home chef, who prepares them with love. Many antique cookbooks include simple recipes for pickling vegetables. You can derive real satisfaction from using these recipes to prepare little jars of your own pickled foods, which will supply regular essential nutrients to your body, especially in winter and early spring.

Experts and enthusiasts say that eating pickled foods helps us get a handle on our sweet tooth, thus protecting our bodies from the harmful effects of sweets. However, we should remember that, despite all the benefits of preparing our vegetables in such a way, we should still consume them in moderation. In the Talmud, one can find a certain bit of wisdom on this topic: "There are three things that are harmful in excess but are beneficial when used sparingly: fermentation, salt and nerves."

We also shouldn't give up cooking our food, since we wouldn't be able to bite, chew, or swallow most foods in their raw state. We just need to know how, so that we don't deprive our food of all its nutrients. Proper, skilled cooking sets off various chemical reactions in our food, making it easier to digest.

Proper meal preparation is not just a culinary art meant to show off the craftsmanship, imagination, taste, and aesthetic sensibilities of yet another master chef but also (and perhaps most important!) knowledge of the fundamental role food plays in our health and lives. We should not only know what we eat but also what is worth eating and what should never touch our lips.

It is possible to make every dish not only an original, beautiful, and appetizing work of culinary art but also a true treasure trove of nutrients that, once eaten, make you want to live and enjoy life to the fullest. Each dish should combine the gifts of nature and the achievements of science in such a way as to preserve the optimal level of nutrients and maximize their use in the human body. I highly recommend a book by Sally Fallon Morell called *Nourishing Traditions: The Cookbook that Challenges Politically Correct Nutrition and the Diet Dictocrats.* Sally is a nutrition journalist and food historian. Her book will teach you to cook correctly, healthily, and deliciously. And it's my favorite!

Synthetic Vitamins: Controversial Copying of Nature

Since 1987, a contender for the title of the eighth wonder of the world can be found on the UNESCO World Heritage List: the Terracotta Army of Qin Shi Huang, the first emperor of China, in the nation's former capital of Xi'an. Each year, two to three million tourists visit the site, where the ruler ordered hundreds of thousands of slaves to make a large, strong, threatening terracotta army near his mausoleum. The army was meant to protect the emperor and his loved ones, guard his treasures, and help the monarch ascend to the throne in the afterlife.

The entire army consists of around eight thousand fired clay figures, who in their life-sized dimensions form a faithful representation of soldiers, officers, medics, and drivers set in battle formation, dressed in uniforms and chain mail and armed with crossbows, spears, and swords. They include foot soldiers, horsemen, and commanders, all ready to engage the enemy at any moment using 130 terracotta chariots, 520 life-sized horses, and a large cavalry.

Each of the clay individuals has his own face and hairstyle (and occasionally mustache), and an expression revealing distinctive emotions. The human and animal figures are dynamic and full of expression. The horses are fired up, with wide-open muzzles, nostrils flared with fury and unease, pricked ears, and windswept manes. When it was first discovered by accident in 1974 by three local farmers digging a well, the army was even more authentic, as it was covered with layers of paint that added realistic emphasis to the figures.

Estimating the site holds around 5,000 more figures, Chinese archeologists continue to work on extracting the mysteries of this site. Experts on the subject, history buffs, and travelers all know that belief in the afterlife is characteristic of many cultures and is a core tenet of numerous religions, while the traditions of building tombs, mausoleums, pyramids, and royal necropolises are timeless and persist in altered forms to this very day.

I'm always amazed by never-ending human attempts to imitate or replace nature, in which unimaginable effort is made to equal or even surpass it and show that we humans are also able to do what it does. The terracotta army was created over a period of thirty years by masses of the greatest craftsmen of the Chinese Empire and anonymous workers of various specialties. It stands as proof of the creative potential of humankind, astounding viewers with its grandeur, precision, and structure.

Yet, it remains an artificial army, a substitute for the real power and ambitious plans of Emperor Qin Shi Huang. Today, the army inspires not only awe but also reflection on humankind's vanity, conviction of its own omnipotence, and desire to compete with the laws of nature.

Everything was precisely copied: weapons, jewelry, caps, mustaches, sandals, harnesses, buckles, combs, and hair adornments—thousands of details that had been observed, that seemed essential, and yet both the people and animals remain mere simulacra, soulless clay mannequins that can only imitate reality. I started to reflect on this rather unexpectedly while working on this chapter on synthetic vitamins and comparing their potential effects with those of their natural counterparts.

Americans spend $22 billion each year on various "life-saving"[208] vitamin supplements meant to work miracles on our bodies and appearance and produced in various forms and configurations. The dietary supplement industry raked in over $32 billion in 2012![209] Is this money well spent? You'll no doubt have your own answer to that question after reading this chapter.

[208] Clement, *Supplements Exposed*, 13.
[209] Derek Beres, "Multivitamins Are Not Only Ineffective but Dangerous," accessed May 20, 2018, http://bigthink.com/21st-century-spirituality/24-billion-later-vitamins-and-supplements-appear-to-have-no-value.

I'll just add one more little thing: statistics show that Americans have the highest incidence rates in the world of many diseases, among which obesity plays an important role. Most of the vitamins currently available on all global markets are synthetically produced in laboratories controlled by pharmaceutical companies, and, as stated by the Organic Consumers Association, as much as 95 percent of them contain synthetic substances having nothing to do with natural sources.[210]

I've already mentioned how many factors work together when the human body uses vitamins. This cooperation is known as synergy. This is a process in which two or more chemical compounds work together to enhance each other's effects, which would be impossible for them to manage by themselves. Synergy is a fundamental principle of nature, but people unfortunately repeatedly ignore it.

Reality shows us that no human could survive on an isolated, synthetic product, because we need healthy and nutritious food created by nature. So far, scientists have been unable to create a real apple from scratch in their laboratories. Only nature has this ability. The scientist Carl Sagan noted humankind's efforts in this regard with the quip "If you wish to make an apple pie from scratch, you must first invent the universe."[211]

---

[210] Adria Vasil, "Organic Consumers Association Takes on the Synthetic Vitamin and Supplements Industry," https://www.organicconsumers.org/news/organic-consumers-association-takes-synthetic-vitamin-and-supplements-industry.

[211] Accessed via https://www.quora.com/What-did-Carl-Sagan-mean-when-he-said-If-you-wish-to-make-apple-pie-from-scratch-you-must-first-create-the-universe.

Michael Pollan answers, "Think about baby formula: we've been working on that one for a century and a half, and for reasons we don't totally understand, it still doesn't do all that genuine mother's milk does. We flatter ourselves by thinking we can outdo or even approximate nature's foods."[212]

When it was proudly announced that artificial sea water could be produced with a chemical makeup identical to that found in real life, it may have seemed that humankind had succeeded in extracting another of nature's closely guarded secrets. As it turns out, saltwater fish introduced to the water either do not survive or survive only in an impaired, weakened condition.

As the online magazine for marine aquarists *Reefkeeping* noted, "The average artificial sea water mix has been recognized for many years as an imperfect substitute for what is the perfect medium for marine animal growth, pure oceanic sea water."[213] As experts maintain, sea water is "a complex and incompletely understood mixture of virtually every substance that has graced the face of the earth."

Humanity's persistence is a beautiful, admirable thing, spurring us to compete with nature and sometimes bringing us great satisfaction but much more often teaching us humility and respect for nature's laws and perfect harmony.

So, what exactly is this natural sea water that has occupied researchers for so long and that holds the only known means of sustaining the rich variety of life in the ocean, generating

[212] M. Pollan, "Answers Readers' Questions," *New York Times Magazine*, October 6, 2011, accessed September 20, 2017, http://michaelpollan.com/articles-archive/michael-pollan-answers-readers-questions/.
[213] R. Shimek, "The Toxicity of Some Freshly Mixed Artificial Sea Water," *Reefkeeping Online*, http://www.reefkeeping.com/issues/2003-03/rs/feature/.

a power that we cannot replicate, no matter how hard we try? The same life force principle that is omnipresent in nature applies here.

The same type of synergy related to the ideal, full range of factors working together (vitamins, minerals, enzymes, coenzymes, bacteria, and hormones) can be found in the healthy, natural food that keeps us alive. This is an extraordinary symphony with countless notes produced by many complicated instruments, which, when played together, create music and become a source of genuine emotion, reflection, and inspiration to act. It seems no true copy can be made.

In his book *Supplements Exposed*, Brian R. Clement states that synthetic vitamins are like the reflection we see in the mirror. The molecules of synthetic and natural vitamins do look the same under a microscope. But just as our reflection cannot actively function on its own but merely imitates our movement, appearance, and expression, so too synthetic vitamins do not work in the same way as their natural, original counterparts. Statistics by the Hippocrates Health Institute in Florida show that 75 percent of people who took synthetic vitamins exhibited symptoms similar to drug or narcotic addiction upon stopping.[214] Most of those studied were healthy people, but synthetic vitamins had a toxic effect on their bodies, nonetheless.

The human body's ability to absorb these vitamins (bioavailability) is seriously hindered. It resembles, perhaps, earthlings' reaction to a potential alien landing, which is not

---

[214] Clement, *Supplements Exposed*, 44.

difficult to imagine. The human body views these vitamins as something alien. It first tries to identify the intruder, so it can then deal with it. Natural vitamins, in contrast, are treated like old friends, which the human corpus has been expecting and welcomes at once, since (like in life) it knows what is natural, authentic, valuable, and necessary. The foreign chemical structure of each unknown element that enters the body must be thoroughly analyzed before it can be used.

Up to 50 percent of a synthetic supplement is treated as something useless that, like waste, should be removed immediately, while the other 50 percent remains something that might eventually come in handy but must first be transformed. Additional resources are needed for this transformation, and these can't be used without incurring internal damage and certain losses. As Marjorie McCullough[215] said in the *New York Times*, "It's possible that the chemicals in the fruits and vegetables on your plate work together in ways that scientists don't fully understand—and which can't be replicated in a tablet."[216]

Nutrients supplied through food don't travel through the human body freely, like aimless drifters in no particular hurry, and they don't just enter our cells, which are waiting in need for them, by accident. Instead, it's as if nutrients contained addresses and postal codes that allowed them to reach cells with the same markings. There's no wandering about, no delays or mistakes. It is a perfect "postal system"

---

[215] Strategic director of nutritional epidemiology for the American Cancer Society.
[216] Liz Szabo, Kaiser Health News, "Older Americans Are 'Hooked' on Vitamins," accessed May 25, 2018, https://www.nytimes.com/2018/04/03/well/older-americans-vitamins-dietary-supplements.html.

developed in our bodies by evolution, and no laboratory-produced synthetic nutrients can compare with its precision, simplicity, speed, or effectiveness. As Dr. Brian R. Clement, director of the Hippocrates Health Institute, notes, "[T]he human biology has never been able to 'digest' synthetic chemicals."[217]

Despite humankind's relatively short history compared to that of the universe, human beings still think they have unlimited potential. Humans may be convinced that they can make the impossible possible but fail to note in their arrogance that both categories are their own, not nature's. This is an incredible attitude—it allows us to believe that we are almighty, omnipotent creators whose every intention is bound to end in success.

This conviction had certainly taken hold in the first emperor of a unified China, at whose command the Great Wall was built and the terracotta army was formed to help him gain power in eternal life. After all, that's why he demanded it be copied so precisely and given the best, most effective, and most realistic weaponry, which allowed him to achieve everything he desired for himself and his dynasty. People found the results of his efforts only in 1974.

Despite the passage of time, the coming of change, and the development of civilization, our attitude toward the world around us, and particularly nature, seems remarkably obdurate and is even typical for a certain segment of today's scientific community.

---

[217] Brian Clement, "Vitamin Myth Exposed," accessed February 6, 2017, https://www.organicconsumers.org/news/nutri-con-truth-about-vitamins-supplements.

To make the issues presented here and their related mechanisms a bit clearer, I'll focus again on the enormously popular vitamin C, which was isolated by the Hungarian physician Albert Szent-Gyorgyi in 1928, winning him a Nobel Prize in 1937. Another figure whose opinions and research led to vitamin C's fame and widespread use is Dr. Linus Pauling, two-time Nobel laureate. He claimed that our ancestors obtained around 600 milligrams of vitamin C a day from their hunting and gathering successes. We should increase this dose, as the quality of food we consume, the state of the environment in which we live, and our rhythm and style of life have seriously declined.

Exhaustive research into vitamin C's functions in the human body interested pharmaceutical companies in synthetic production of the vitamin. The research results were used in intensive advertising campaigns, but any negative research indications of the significantly divergent effects of natural and synthetic vitamin C were systematically silenced or avoided.

Vitamin C is one of the most important agents eliminating toxins from the human body, especially carcinogenic nitrosamines, which are a by-product of heat-treating food (e.g., curing meats) or arise spontaneously in stored food products. The *Tufts University Health and Nutrition Letter* reports that synthetic vitamin C does not exhibit these properties.[218] Even food-derived vitamin C ceases to be effective at detoxifying our bodies, as it has been deprived of its support in the form of bioflavonoids. These are essential to activating vitamin C, since they reduce capillary fragility and permeability.

---

[218]   Randall Fitzgerald, *The Hundred-Year Lie: How Food and Medicine Are Destroying Your Health* (New York: Penguin Group, 2006), 282.

The dietician Dr. Laura Mason-Scarborough illustrates the differences between natural and synthetic vitamin C with the simple and clear argument "What do you get if you purchase a synthesized bottle of vitamin C? You are buying ascorbic acid, a small part of vitamin C, manufactured from super-refined corn sugar. Ascorbic acid does have strong effects on the body but is more of a drug than a nutrient."[219]

Laboratory-produced vitamin C offers limited bioavailability and only some of the beneficial immune system effects compared with that found in natural sources. You can provide arguments for this thesis yourself by doing a simple experiment. When you notice a cold coming on, consume some amla berry extract (in the amount recommended on the packaging), for example. This is a fruit native to Asia that is very rich in vitamin C. Known in India since ancient times and also called amalaki or Indian gooseberry, it is famous for slowing the aging process, providing strength, and fighting numerous illnesses. As it turns out, all this is thanks to the whopping 720 milligrams of vitamin C found in every 100 grams of the raw product!

As Hippocrates stressed, "If it's possible to cure with nature, look to nature first." So, I also recommend camu camu (camo camo, cacari), the fruit of a shrub native to the Amazon. Camu camu fruit are lime-sized and orange to red in color and are available dried in health food stores. They are exceptionally rich in vitamin C, containing 1,800 to 2,500 milligrams for every 100 grams of flesh. Camu camu is known as the ambrosia of the Amazon.

---

[219] Laura Manson-Scarborough, "Synthetic or Natural Vitamins—What's the Difference?" last updated October 16, 2008, https://www.healthychild.com/synthetic-or-natural-vitamins-whats-the-difference/.

As for natural vitamin C content, however, camu camu still comes in second to the Kakadu plum (*Terminalia ferdinandiana*) of Australia. The undisputed leader in this regard, this fruit boasts 3,200 to 5,000 milligrams of vitamin C per 100 grams! You can also use acerola berries (wild crepe myrtle or Barbados cherry), which have a slightly lower vitamin C content of 1,400 to 2,500 milligrams per 100 grams of fruit, or bee pollen, which is available at pharmacies or natural food stores.

When you decide to use any one of these natural wellsprings of vitamin C at the onset of a cold, carefully observe and record how you feel. The next time you feel a sniffle coming on, take some synthetic vitamin C and keep close track of what happens. Write your observations down again and compare them to your previous ones. I've done exactly that, and the difference is enormous! Now, nobody can talk me into taking synthetic vitamin C and introducing something like that to my body again!

The differences can be seen not only in the divergent effects of vitamin C in the living body but also in the way it is obtained. This is easy to follow in the case of amla berries. When producing complete vitamin C from these fruits, first the inedible husk and cellulose are removed, and then the berries' pulp is rinsed with water, ground up, and dried at low temperatures, allowing them to retain all their nutrients and the biological factors that work with them. No freezing technology is used, nor are the berries subject to additional chemical nutritional enhancement.

Meanwhile, synthetics are made in a laboratory from corn sugar or coal tar, which are the foundational substances of synthetic vitamin supplements.[220] Added to these are aspartame (in effervescent tablets, for example) and pigments, such as titanium dioxide, a suspected carcinogen; artificial FD&C Blue No. 2; aluminum lake; and FD&C Red No. 40. They also often contain sucrose, citric acid monohydrate, sodium benzoate, cochineal red (E124), brilliant black (E151), and sometimes artificial flavors as well. We get a product that is long-lasting, colorful, fragrant, in attractive packaging, and ... I'll leave the rest up to you.

Natural vitamins are fortunately devoid of such attractions. When consumed with healthy food, they can work miracles in our bodies. For example, an article appearing in the *Journal of Orthomolecular Medicine* describes in detail how antioxidants and vitamins work together to fight free radicals.[221] They work systematically and with precision, as a well-coordinated team—a perfect example of natural synergy. When vitamin E neutralizes reactive oxygen species (ROS), it becomes oxidized itself. To deal the final blow to ROS, it must return to its original form as vitamin E, which it does thanks to the help of vitamin C or glutathione.

To finish our discussion, I'd like to quote Dr. Jeffrey Blumberg, nutrition specialist and director of the well-known Antioxidants Laboratory at the Human Nutrition Research Center in Boston. He gave this opinion during an interview on CNN: "There are about 20,000 different antioxidants in our diet. There aren't 20,000 different pills to take. One of the reasons dietary supplements can't replace a healthful diet

---

[220] Clement, *Supplements Exposed*, 50.
[221] J. J. Challem, "Beta-Carotene and Other Carotenoids: Promises, Failures and a New Vision," *Journal of Orthomolecular Medicine* 12 (1997).

is because we don't know about what's important to put in every pill."[222]

If our soil is depleted of its nutrients and poisoned with dangerous chemical waste, pesticides, weed killers, and insecticides and our environment is industrially devastated, even while the vitamins we find on supermarket or pharmacy shelves poison us rather than help and strengthen us— what should we do *not only to survive* but live healthily and responsibly despite it all? We've got to rekindle a bit of our longing for authentic, genuine contact with *Mother Nature* and reestablish this contact as best as we can!

Start with the simplest things. I suggest you buy a large wicker basket and, first thing in the morning, march straight to your local market[223] for fresh fruits and vegetables. You've got to change your attitude toward meal preparation. This can be a time of real artistic creation, a valuable time that is just for us. You can also invite friends and loved ones to join you. Pamper yourself and your family with wonderful food this way, win sincere compliments, learn new recipes, take satisfaction from your successful attempts, and decorate the dishes you serve.

In every country, everywhere in the world, there are regional markets where you can find local farmers, gardeners, fruit farmers, and breeders selling their products. My advice is to *befriend them*!

---

[222] Caleb Hellerman, "No Scientific Evidence Diet Supplements Work," CNN 2007, http://edition.cnn.com/2007/HEALTH/04/06/chasing.supplements/.

[223] For busy people or people who do not have a farmer's market in the nearest neighborhood, our modern times offer an excellent opportunity to order farmer's products straight from the farmer via the Internet.

I do my shopping at an organic farmer's market every Tuesday and Saturday. I love these days and eagerly await them, getting up quite early to avoid traffic and to not have trouble finding a parking space. I love these shopping adventures! Weaving my way contentedly through the stalls full of fresh, fragrant, colorful products, I exuberantly select the highest-quality vegetables, fruit, herbs, dairy, eggs, fish, nuts, honey, homemade butter, and so on. I breathe in and savor the wonderful aroma of early strawberries, tomatoes, and peppers. Then, I buy bunches of flowers for my home and seedlings for my patio. I'm completely in my element! I happily haul my basketful of wonderful spoils, my vitamin and mineral marvels!

The sellers and I warmly greet one another. Everybody knows everybody at my market, and everyone knows me. They offer me true delicacies, since they can tell that I respect and admire their work, and I know how much effort they put into their harvest. I select a shiny apple and remember that it can't be made from scratch in any laboratory in the world. I remember, before it crunches delightfully as I bite into it and then melts in my mouth, it was created and worked on for years by the power of nature and these people's labor, patience, love, and care.

Without all this, my and my family's health and well-being would be difficult to attain. Happy to spend my money on these farmer's markets' products, I hope that these small farms, gardens, orchards, and plots will be able to prosper and support the farmers and their families for years to come. I believe that we will all benefit from it, including me and my family.

Nothing can take the place of a fresh meal of salads; cooked, pickled, or raw vegetables; nutritious protein; and healthy fat. I've often noted a certain Protestant reaction against spending money on such "luxury" food. Curiously, this frugality doesn't extend to other indulgences, such as fancy apartments, sports cars, designer clothes, and so on. But if you think clearly and logically, the amount spent on quality food at a market is far less than what you would end up shelling out to cover doctor's bills and treatment after getting sick or less than any loss of income from losing your job.

Our food should be varied, since only then does it provide all the nutrients we need. To do so, we need fresh products, honest desire, a bit of ingenuity, and sometimes a good cookbook or family recipe that's been passed down for generations! A healthy diet is never about perfection; it's always about practice.

I also assure you that cooking meals, setting the table, and sitting down to lunch or dinner together are all wonderful occasions for conversation, reflection, planning, and simply opening up to others, and they help build warm and close relationships in your household.

You can't even imagine my excitement and delight when I come home from the market on Saturday morning, unpack my colorful and delicious trophies on the table, and then fill up the fridge and the fruit bowl and finally put together the ultimate breakfast for my loved ones. How much joy my family's happy, still-sleepy faces give me as they appear in the dining room, enticed by the smell of fresh, organic coffee with cream straight from the farm and the aroma of breakfast sitting on the table—only those who have shared this pleasure with us can know! In short, *I just love these mornings!*

Don't think that I slave away for hours in the kitchen, either. Nothing of the sort! For me, preparing meals is not a sacrifice or some unpleasant, tiresome duty. I can do it easily and quickly, since my meals are not only tasty and healthy but also easy to make and don't require too much time. [224]

Minerals in the Microworld of the Human Body

Bioelements, like vitamins, are present in every nutritious food Mother Nature gives us. They are vital to our health, proper functioning, development, and well-being and a normal reproductive process. These elements enter our food from the soil in which plants are grown.

We can distinguish seven basic minerals that we need to support the fundamental functions of the human body's cells and tissues:

- calcium
- chlorine
- potassium
- magnesium
- phosphorus
- sodium
- sulfur

---

[224] Take a look at my website, where you can find many interesting, healthy recipes, cooking tips, and tutorials. My next publication dedicated to the art of healthy cooking will be coming out shortly. I believe that the book will meet the expectations of those interested in sensible, organic, and healthy cuisine.

In addition to these, nearly all the elements that appear in nature can be found in our organic microworld. We've got nearly all of Mendeleev's periodic table inside us!

Of course, these elements appear in varying amounts, which is why they go by different names. Trace elements are also known as microelements, over thirty of which have been recognized by experts as being essential to life and maintaining good health. Besides such well-known elements as iron, iodine, zinc, and copper, our bodies also need other, less-popular but no less important ones like cobalt, boron, germanium, silicon, fluoride, lithium, selenium, and so on.

We obtain these elements in many different forms but most often through food, water, and salt. The mineral content of our food and our bodies, in turn, depend on their presence in the soil in which the plants we eat are grown. Of course, industrial and chemical degradation of the soil has led to its depletion and contamination, making it impossible to raise plants that would ensure an optimal supply of the minerals we need. Only the renewal of our farmland and a return to organic methods of food production can restore the necessary minerals in our food.

The use of chemicals in the form of pesticides, herbicides, and artificial fertilizers is now widespread, but it was introduced to mass agriculture only relatively recently (in the nineteenth and twentieth centuries). Chemical fertilization was introduced in the mid-nineteenth century by the German scientist Justus von Liebig. In all likelihood, he never thought his idea for enriching the soil would end up impoverishing it. When exploited to the limit, farmland becomes barren and mineral-poor, making it utterly impossible for it to transfer the minerals we need into the plants growing in it.

Real, wholesome food should be grown in healthy soil that is full of minerals and living organisms. Strong plants can deal naturally with any inhospitable climate conditions and pests. Consuming food produced this way influences our physical condition and health, ensuring our vitality and proper bodily functioning. Such food also boosts the immune system, making it more effective against viruses and bacteria and guaranteeing a higher quality of life and work.

Every cell in the complex human microworld benefits from this. In this sphere, millions of physiological processes take place twenty-four hours a day, and among other things, they require an appropriate level of minerals. For us to enjoy this blessing, our farmland must first regain its original morphology and full potential. This is an absolute prerequisite for the health of contemporary humans and future generations.

As the spiritual occupants of our organic home, we should live comfortably within it, without making forced renovations, threats, or unnecessary expenditures.

The German chemist Justus von Liebig, mentioned earlier, studied the influence of environmental factors on living organisms. He is the discoverer and creator of the law of the minimum. According to von Liebig, the scarcest factor in an environment is the one that limits the growth and functioning of a given organism.

This is also true for the human body. Supplying the right amounts of essential minerals to our bodies is incredibly important, since every deficit negatively affects our health. Minerals like zinc, copper, and magnesium work as mediators and are crucial factors that operate together and determine whether vitamins are effective or not. In the same way, the presence of vitamins is necessary for minerals to be absorbed. Vitamin D, for example, is required for proper calcium absorption, while vitamin C is needed to absorb iron, especially when that iron comes from plant sources. Copper is required to activate vitamin C.

Mineral deficiencies are generally also a sign of vitamin deficiencies in the body. The human body can use itself as a source of these minerals for a certain period of time if they're not supplied by our food, drawing upon various parts of itself, i.e., our bones, liver, and muscles. Our system is built so that our bloodstream must be in balance. If this equilibrium is upset, then "autocannibalism" occurs: the body literally begins to consume itself.

Our vitality crucially depends on minerals. They make up 4 percent of our body weight, with trace elements comprising 0.01 percent. Around 2 percent of our body weight is due to minerals found in the solid parts of the human body: bones, teeth, nails, hair, and soft tissue. The remainder is found in our fluids: in the blood, interstitial fluid, and intracellular fluid. Keep in mind, as much as 80 percent of our weight is water.

Minerals are our vital energy and must be consumed daily for our bodies to function properly. They control our metabolic processes, maintain the physical and chemical integrity of our cells and tissues, and determine which enzymatic reactions occur.

There's an enormous difference between organic minerals, derived from living organisms, and inorganic ones. Organic minerals come from animals or plants and are found in units of living or recently living matter. Organic minerals— bioelements—are mainly provided by plant-based food or by drinking vegetable and bone broth that has been cooked for several hours and in which all the macroelements (calcium, chlorine, magnesium, phosphorus, sodium, sulfur, and potassium) are ready to be consumed and are easily assimilated by the body.

Vegetable root systems can change the properties of the unnatural materials they convert into useful, organic ones.[225] Inorganic minerals do not come from plant or animal sources but are obtained from rock, sand, chalk, and inanimate shells (e.g., eggshells, seashells, carapaces, and so on). They are not food and are in fact very harmful to us.

Our bodies do not recognize such minerals as food, even if they once were alive and became fossilized over millions of years. More and more scientific evidence shows that adding synthetic minerals and toxic nutritional supplements to human food is worse over the long term for our health than completely giving them up. Consumers of such products should proceed with extreme caution and look closely at the information provided on the labels to be sure that the vitamins or minerals offered come from a "living" source. The human body requires real, organically raised food to stay in good condition and gain strength and energy. As the simple and clear saying goes, "Life needs life to stay alive."

There are many elements that appear alongside and work together with the organic minerals found in wholesome food.

---

[225] The word *organic*, meanwhile, is often overused. It is a term referring to minerals and some chemical compounds, not "living" beings, which can cause confusion.

These include enzymes, vitamins, hormones, oxygen, nitrogen, and many other still-unknown components that work in concert and whose functions and participation in many processes are still waiting to be discovered. As with vitamins, nature has yet to create isolated minerals unaccompanied by other elements playing the role of cofactors. We know, however, that it is not so much the mineral in its pure form that is of decisive significance but the other elements that come with it.

All this makes the natural form of the mineral more effective than—and incomparable to—any other form. The minerals found in organic food are also naturally chelated units (i.e., changed into a form that is easy for the human body to remove), which effortlessly combine with other minerals, vitamins, oxygen, or many other elements. Chlorophyll binds a magnesium atom, hemoglobin binds iron, and, along with enzymes, they chelate copper, iron, zinc, and manganese.

The example of alfalfa, a member of the pea family with the highest nutritional value of any sprout, is a good illustration of the mechanisms of this process. The plant absorbs calcium carbonate from the soil, which is then metabolized by its natural chemical processing plant into calcium phytate or other calcium compounds.

In addition, many vitamins and minerals must be combined with this compound so that this one-of-a-kind source of a naturally occurring, unique calcium complex can be formed. Therefore, providing isolated calcium or synthetic calcium is not enough. After all, the essential elements that appear in organic conditions do not cooperate with this form. Only when consumed together do they fulfill their proper role in our bodies. In short, the calcium that is absorbed by the plant must first be processed by its unique chemical processing unit into a form that is readily absorbed and then easily digested by the human body in turn.

However, this process doesn't always go off without a hitch. There are many factors that can block mineral absorption. This happens even when these minerals are present in our food. The system of glands responsible for sending signals to the intestinal mucosa requires vast reserves of fat-soluble vitamins (A, D, E, and K) to work properly and effectively.

The intestinal mucosa itself needs these vitamins along with sufficient cholesterol. This is due to the need to maintain intestinal cohesion, so that only those nutrients the body needs are absorbed. The body must also remain impenetrable to unsafe toxins and large, undigested proteins, which may cause allergic reactions or other pathological complications. Minerals wanting to enter our cells may "compete" for receptor space. Too much calcium clearly hinders manganese absorption. A lack of hydrochloric acid in the stomach, an alkaline environment in the intestines, a deficiency in certain enzymes, and an insufficient amount of vitamin C or other nutrients can prevent chelates from releasing minerals from their "pincer-like" bonds (the Greek *chele* means a crab's pincers or claws). Antinutritional factors can also block absorption by binding ionized minerals in the GI tract. These harmful agents include phytic acid in grains, oxalic acid in green vegetables, and tannins in tea.

Of course, knowing a few fundamental facts about macro- and microelements and their deficiency or excess in the human body will play an important role in our lives and decisions regarding the quality and structure of our diet, based on our individual needs.

Remember

- Synthetic vitamins are deprived of the minerals, bioflavonoids, phenols, and other phytonutrients that always work together with natural vitamins, so that they can exert their greatest effects.
- Taking synthetic supplements carries the risk of consuming toxic dyes, preservatives, artificial flavors, and harmful sweeteners.
- The best minerals for our bodies are organic minerals obtained from a healthy, varied diet.
- Too many or too few bioelements can set off harmful processes in the human body and cause many dangerous, even life-threatening illnesses.
- Two easily available and rich sources of many minerals are unrefined sea salt and bone broth.
- Adding crystals of natural, unrefined mined salt or sea salt to salads or water is an excellent way to make up for bioelement losses caused by intense work, physical exertion, a hectic lifestyle, stress, or heat waves.
- If you follow a proper diet, drink lots of good quality water, exercise, and take time to rest and sleep, then you can add some good quality natural supplements if you still need them—but not the other way around! As they say, "It doesn't matter if you use golden nails; a boat made of rotten wood will only sink, taking your golden nails right to the bottom."

CHAPTER 14

ENZYMES: ÉMINENCE GRISE OF YOUR METABOLISM

Obtaining food from outside sources is a fundamental prerequisite of existence for every living organism. However, if these nutrients are not properly processed and absorbed, this can have much more serious consequences than occasional discomfort or slight hiccups in our health. Of course, what is true for every living organism is also true for the human body. Only a robust, well-functioning digestive system can ensure the body's optimal condition, development, and functioning, since only then is it able to mechanically and chemically process the food it receives.

Apart from water, simple sugars, and mineral salts, which our bodies can absorb without any further processing, every organic compound must be broken down into simple substances so that it can be processed smoothly. This interdependent, complex chain of mechanical and chemical changes to our food is what we call digestion. Our food's components reach every living cell in our bodies thanks to this process. The mechanical stage of food processing includes grinding and chewing, swallowing, and transport through the different segments of our GI tract. The chemical stage is possible because of digestive enzymes produced by the human body (also known as digestive juices or, historically, digestive ferments).

Of course, eating the healthiest, most nutritious food is all for naught if our GI tract and entire digestive system fail us. Enzymes play an important role in this network of complex digestive processes.

The food in our mouths is a diverse mix of organic macromolecules. It includes fats, proteins, and carbohydrates, along with vitamins, minerals, and many other elements. For all of them to make it into our blood and then become valuable building blocks for creating, rebuilding, and repairing our cells or become a source of energy necessary for our inner organs to function or provide the right resources to our bodies, these macromolecules must first be broken down into smaller molecules, and then further into chemical substances that the body can recognize and happily absorb.

Fortunately, the reliable and precise course of evolution has built a highly sophisticated system to achieve this. As we slowly chew our last bite of food, digestive enzymes are released. The large macromolecules are then broken down into easily assimilated smaller components in both the stomach and the small intestine (via the liver, pancreas, and gallbladder). These organic compounds are absorbed with water and mineral salts through the lining of the GI tract and enter the body's blood and lymph fluids. Thanks to these fluids, the compounds travel to every cell and tissue, where they are assimilated and used to complete their tasks programmed by nature.

Nutritional researchers discovered enzymes in the twentieth century, around the same time as vitamins and minerals. However, the first signs of their existence appeared in 1876, in research German scientist Wilhelm Friedrich Kühne conducted. Enzymes are complex proteins that act as catalysts in nearly every biochemical process in all living organisms, as well as viruses.

Their level of activity depends on the presence of the right vitamins and minerals. Many enzymes contain only a single molecule of trace minerals, such as copper, iron, or zinc, without which these enzymes couldn't function. In the 1930s, biochemists proudly announced that around eighty such enzymes had been discovered, with more to come. Today, we know of over five thousand—and we're still counting.

Enzymes are classified into three basic groups, with numerous subgroups. The largest group is the *metabolic enzymes*, which play an important role in physiological processes like breathing, talking, moving, thinking, behavior, and immune system maintenance. A subgroup of these enzymes is responsible for neutralizing toxins and carcinogenic pollutants, such as DDT and tobacco smoke, by changing them into less-toxic forms that the body can then eliminate.

The second category is the digestive enzymes, of which only twenty-two have been found so far. Most are produced by the pancreas, but there are some made by glands in the duodenum. Their job is to process food that has been partially digested and released by the stomach.

The enzymes that we must consider as we plan our diet are those belonging to the third group: food enzymes. They are present in raw food and initiate the digestive process in the mouth and upper stomach.

They are assigned strictly specialized tasks in the human body:

- Protease is an enzyme that helps digest different kinds of proteins.
- Lipases are a general class of enzymes that break down fat molecules (lipids).
- Amylase is a digestive enzyme that acts on starch in food, breaking it down into smaller carbohydrate molecules.

Enzymes found in food continue these processes as the food reaches the stomach and comes to a stop in its upper part. No digestive juices are released here, as this section functions similarly to a bird's stomach or the first stomach of ruminant animals. The upper human stomach is like a container in which the enzymes in raw foods can perform their tasks and partially process what we've consumed into a smooth, homogeneous mass.

Once in this form, our food can easily move on to the lower parts of our GI tract. Hydrochloric acid is released only in the lower part of the stomach and is stimulated by food traveling from the upper to the lower part. Once in the stomach, it goes to work, disinfecting and triggering the breakdown of food. One thing many people don't know is that hydrochloric acid doesn't digest meat on its own. Instead, it transforms the enzyme pepsinogen into its active form, pepsin. The pepsin then breaks down the proteins found in meat and turns it into more easily digestible soluble proteins called peptones.

Research on enzymes has shown that, while they work on a certain class of organic compounds, they are chemically neutral toward others, and their level of chemical activity is determined by the temperature and pH of their environment. It has also revealed the significance of raw food in our diet and how important the enzymes that such food contains are, since they start up the initial stage of digestion and relieve the body of the need to produce additional digestive enzymes.

Temperatures over 65°C (150°F) destroy enzymes. The optimal temperature for enzyme functioning fluctuates between 37°C and 40°C (98.6°F and 104°F). Some are active in a neutral environment (pH = 7), while others only become active in an acidic (pH < 7) or basic (alkaline) environment.

A diet consisting exclusively of cooked foods puts a heavy burden on the pancreas and strains its ability to participate in the digestive process. If the pancreas is constantly forced to produce enzymes that have been removed from food at high temperatures, it becomes weakened over time. People who eat a diet of mainly cooked foods put excessive strain on their pancreas and other digestive organs.

Such actions have serious repercussions. According to the late Dr. Edward Howell, a pioneer in enzyme research, these consequences could include a shortened life span, illness, and lower resistance to all types of stress. He noted that humans and animals whose diet was primarily made up of cooked foods demonstrate an enlarged pancreas, while other organs and glands—particularly the brain—actually shrink.[226]

---

[226] Edward Howell, *Enzymes for Health and Longevity* (Woodstock Valley: Omangod Press, 1980).

His research also showed that the human body recycles enzymes by absorbing them through the walls of the intestines or colon and transporting them in the blood back to the upper intestines. There, they are used again. The human body has been built economically by nature: nothing valuable is wasted, and so it protects its valuable enzyme reserves.

Doctor Howell formulated the following axiom: "The length of life is inversely proportional to the rate of exhaustion of the enzyme potential of an organism. The increased use of food enzymes promotes a decreased rate of exhaustion of the enzyme potential."[227]

Another principle can be expressed as follows: nutritious, unprocessed, raw food is the foundation for good health. Such food not only provides the full range of valuable enzymes that enable numerous chemical processes to run properly during digestion, but it is also a source of unlimited natural energy and vitality.

The cuisines of nearly all traditional societies feature dishes containing raw, enzyme-rich products. For example, consider the following:

- Sauerkraut is an excellent source of enzymes and living probiotics.
- Avocado contains lipase, a fat-digesting enzyme that is essential in the metabolism of fats.
- Pineapple contains papain, an enzyme that breaks down proteins into amino acids so we can utilize them to aid in the healing and growth of our bodies.

---

[227] Edward Howell, *Enzyme Nutrition* (USA: Avery Publishing Group, 1985).

These traditional dishes include not only plant-based foods but also raw animal proteins, fats from unprocessed dairy foods, raw meat, animal organs, and fish. The dishes made from these ingredients include a variety of natural bacterial cultures and, of course, many groups of priceless enzymes that make fermentation or bacterial culture growth possible.

For example, the Inuit have a singular way of preparing fish in which they allow fresh fish to "spoil," as they know that this "predigests" the fish. Some Asian cultures couldn't imagine preparing a meal without fish sauce, which is produced from fish that have been allowed to "rot" in barrels in the open air. This sauce is highly prized in their cuisine (although it does stink to high heaven), and adding it regularly to all their soups and sauces, perhaps surprisingly, improves their taste.

The fermentation of various dairy products has been practiced for thousands of years in even the most ancient cultures. This process increases the enzyme content of milk, cream, butter, and cheeses. Ethnic groups whose diet is based on cooked meat usually supplement their enzyme reserves with fermented products, such as sauerkraut, pickles, kvass, borscht, and "white borscht" made from fermented rye.

Japan's venerable *miso* and *natto*—foods made from fermented soybeans with the addition of rice or barley and yeast—may scare off more sensitive consumers with their unusual smell (offensive to some) but are widely prized sources of enzymes when consumed unheated. Raw meat that has been rubbed with marjoram[228] a few hours before being consumed is more easily digested by the human body.

---

[228] Marjoram keeps meat fresh longer.

Grains, nuts, and legumes contain many valuable enzymes, but these cannot be fully used by consumers because of enzyme inhibitors. Soaking these foods in acidic or salted water or fermenting them deactivates these inhibitors. Nearly all fruits and vegetables contain enzymes, but these are even more sensitive to high and low temperatures than vitamins are. Cooking, pasteurization, and freezing all damage them. Such enzymes are most active around the human body's natural temperature.

Extra virgin olive oil and other unrefined oils; natural, unrefined honey; grapes; figs; avocados; bananas; papayas; pineapples; kiwis; and mangoes are highly recommended as part of your daily diet, since they are exceptionally rich in these biocatalysts, which regulate the vital processes taking place in the human body so well.

The principle of the golden mean, known since ancient times, is also useful when planning a healthy diet. Stoic restraint would have us remember that there is no known, traditional diet based entirely on raw food, even though there are raw foodists and fruitarians who would like to convince us otherwise.

We should eat raw food daily for many reasons (already discussed in this book), but it should be in the right proportion to the rest of our diet. Even in tropical regions, where lighting a fire during the day is not necessary to warm one's body or dwelling, the custom and need to construct primitive fireplaces for preparing heat-treated meals have existed since the most ancient times.

Some nutrients are more accessible and more easily released from our food through cooking. The high temperatures of a direct flame or boiling water can neutralize some toxins and kill health-threatening microorganisms. Generally, cereal bran, grains, beans, cabbage, and many other vegetables should be cooked, while animal products should be eaten both cooked and raw.

Of course, we should chew everything carefully, so that our salivary amylase (ptyalin) permeates every bite of food, softens it, allows it to be coated in saliva for easier swallowing, and forms a more viscous pulp, preventing dry crumbs from entering the respiratory tract. Saliva, which contains ptyalin, starts up the process of converting polysaccharides into disaccharides. The human body produces 1 to 1.5 liters of saliva each day.

Thorough, slow chewing also brings our food to the right temperature, making further digestion easier. Though it may sound funny, the Talmud saying still rings true: "Chew well with your teeth, and you will find it in your legs." This expression shows a certain appreciation for this initial metabolic process that takes place as soon as our food reaches our mouths.

When I mentioned moderation and its role in a proper diet, I had in mind not only an appropriate amount and quality of food but also suitable proportions of raw and cooked food. Meat should always be consumed along with fresh, raw, or fermented vegetables, especially their green parts (parsley, chives, dill, kale, celery, cilantro, and leeks). This is not only to preserve their active enzymes but also because of their fiber, which is crucial to the digestive process and serves as food for the "good" bacteria in our gut.

Experts warn against a completely raw diet, since the key to optimal health lies in the variety of foods we eat, moderation, reason, and knowledge. As a personal example, I know someone who, after eight months of following a strict raw food diet, landed in the hospital with severe anemia, her hair falling out in clumps. I also know a person who has eaten raw and vegan food for years and looks physically healthy.

Reduced digestive enzyme reserves are one of the causes of gastrointestinal dysfunction. Other reasons for a decrease in enzymes include the following:

- incorrect proportions of carbohydrates, fats, and protein in the diet
- an insufficient intake of natural vitamins and minerals (i.e., a diet poor in raw foods)
- bad eating habits—eating on the run, incomplete chewing, greedily swallowing big, dry bites of food
- the presence of artificial dyes, flavors, and preservatives in industrially processed food
- excess refined carbohydrates in the diet
- age—after age forty, the loss of enzymes in the body is almost unavoidable, amounting to a loss of a third of our reserves compared to those at age twenty
- consuming very hot or very cold foods; in these conditions, sensitive enzymes are damaged more quickly than vitamins

Today, more and more factors are starting to contribute to the depletion or weakening of these beneficial substances. To bring our devastated and enzyme-depleted GI tract back to normal and to help it function properly, we should take a few simple, tried-and-true preventative measures. Fortunately, we can add several more foods to the list of raw and fermented products already mentioned, and it should all start with … the first bite.

- *Chew your food calmly and fully.* Today's world is in such a rush that we easily forget where we're hurrying to and why. As we live at such a hectic pace, many things escape our notice, since they're so obvious and normal that we assume they can't be worth worrying about. I don't suggest you treat your food this way or ignore the environment and conditions in which you eat it. When we savor the simple pleasures of life, in the words of Mother Teresa, "holiness is something we experience each day." We should keep this idea in mind and not only at the table. I am deeply convinced that nothing compares to the satisfaction of sharing even the simplest meal with family and friends, with whom we can savor and discuss the taste, aroma, and appearance of the food we're enjoying. The brain stem sends out stimuli to release stomach acid and prepare enzymes to process food at the mere thought of our meal, not to mention the food's appearance, aroma, the table setting, and so on. All of this awakens our senses and readies our digestive systems. There are various reasons—not only emotional and aesthetic but especially physiological—to take the time to thoroughly chew our food. It's certainly not time wasted. This is time invested in our health! First, slowly chewing our food transforms our bites of food into a liquefied substance, which greatly aids digestion. Secondly, calm chewing stimulates the production of saliva, which contains the necessary enzymes and prepares this substance to be safely swallowed. This makes our food ready to move on to the next stage of processing in the stomach and small intestine. Thirdly, this process stimulates the parotid glands, which release hormones that trigger T cell production in the thyroid. These cells play a crucial role in maintaining our immune system. Fourthly, this ideal method of chewing stimulates the pancreas and other digestive organs. Chewing is a wonderfully designed component of the automated communication system, keeping the organs in the human corpus working in perfect harmony. Don't disrupt this ideal mechanism of cooperation by omitting the important first step—chew completely!

• *Avoid chewing gum.* This ubiquitous and widely consumed product is a dangerous, deceitful vandal that wreaks havoc and confusion in our digestive system! Chewing gum disrupts the coordinated reactions of our digestive system presented earlier. Each time we begin to chew, our brain thinks that we're starting to eat. In response, it sends a signal to the stomach, pancreas, and other digestive organs to get ready for digestion. Following the brain's orders, the pancreas begins to needlessly (and unfortunately!) overproduce enzymes that are then wasted, since they won't be used in any chemical process. This natural source of enzymes has its limits! If these false signals are repeated often enough, the gland is weakened by this repeated, senseless effort. It's easy to imagine how, in such a condition, the pancreas wouldn't be able to produce enough enzymes when real food is consumed. Nobody can drink from a dried-up source.

o   One solution for replenishing our digestive juices could be …

- *Supplement enzymes.* I've already indicated many times that I'm not a fan of supplements as a way of supplying nutrients for the human body's overall development and functioning. But as the old saying goes, sometimes the exception proves the rule. You'll soon see how even a small deviation from the accepted rules can sometimes be enormously helpful. High-quality enzyme supplements can broaden the range of benefits we'd like to derive from a good meal. Troublesome bloating, minor stomach problems, unpleasant burping, occasional constipation, and many other unwelcome surprises take the pleasure out of eating and significantly limit our selection of nutritious foods—after all, we'd like to eat them but are forced give many of them up to avoid these problems. This is where enzyme supplements should come in, since they can free us from these dilemmas. These supplements must be of the highest quality to guarantee the intended results. Taking such enzymes during a meal is like hiring an additional backup unit, allowing you to speed up, simplify, improve, and streamline important tasks without using additional, precious energy. Every employer dreams of having such a contractor at hand when previous efforts have proved insufficient! Today, you can purchase any type of enzyme, from those that help digest proteins and carbohydrates to specialized enzymes for people with a lactose or gluten intolerance. However, I will continue to tirelessly stress that supplements cannot take the place of healthy, fresh, natural food.

From the preceding, we can see that the threat to our health and lives doesn't just come from an industrialized environment but also (to a greater degree and more insidiously) from conventional farming methods that wreak chemical devastation on both the soil and crops. Seeking only profit, these farms contaminate their local biosystems with excessive use of artificial fertilizers and protective agents. The soil becomes depleted of all the elements we need, such as copper, iron, and magnesium and in their place appear unsafe levels of minerals that are toxic or even lethal to humans. Unfortunately, crops raised in such conditions exhibit the same characteristics.

Our bodies' evolutionary defense mechanisms can deal with most of these negative circumstances only if we arm our "natural bodyguards" with the proper nutritional weapons in our food. Minerals like calcium and magnesium, as well as antioxidants such as vitamin A, carotene, vitamin C, vitamin E, and selenium protect us against heavy metals and remove substantial amounts of such toxins from our bodies. Proper silicon levels provide excellent protection against aluminum, while zinc effectively fights off toxic cadmium.

So where should we get these effective, reliable "weapons" for our army of protectors? An organic, balanced diet solves this problem beautifully. Making sure we get only the highest quality food and water as well as meticulous inspection of the products we buy are absolute musts if we want to guarantee our optimal health as well as complete physical and mental fitness. Such behavior allows us to consciously and effectively eliminate many harmful, even life-threatening substances. Getting your food from reliable sources, avoiding highly processed products, or asking for information on ingredients and sources in dishes are not all part of some frivolous, irritating fad but together form a responsible attitude to your health that reflects the seriousness of the problem—we're talking about our most valuable assets here, *our health and lives!*

Let's boycott those businesses, companies, and restaurants that fail to respect this attitude, where attempts to find out this essential information are either ignored or dismissed as mere eccentricity (or worse).

Remember

- Enzymes are essential for the complex digestive processes in the body to run properly.
- Raw, healthy food is a natural source of a variety of valuable enzymes.

- A diet rich in animal protein should always be accompanied by appropriate amounts of raw or fermented products that are rich in fiber and enzymes.
- Highly processed food has been stripped of many essential nutrients, including beneficial enzymes.
- Chewing our food thoroughly allows it to mix with the enzymes found in our saliva and is an important stage in the digestive process.
- The enzymes in the body create the right conditions for the development of essential, helpful bacterial cultures in our GI tract, which eliminate pathogens and support the digestive process.
- We should give up chewing gum once and for all.
- High-quality enzyme supplements can be used to counteract enzyme deficiencies in our diet.

CHAPTER 15

MEDICATION, USED RESPONSIBLY

Disease and diagnosis as we know it will soon be an obsolete concept, an artifact of medical history, like bloodletting or phrenology (the art of diagnosis based on the shape of your skull, popular in the 19th century). The reason is simply this: Naming a disease does nothing to help us identify and treat the underlying causes of the disease. We must address these causes if we have any hope of helping individuals heal … We have to think about individuals, not diseases. In medicine, our genetic differences are more important than our similarities.
—Dr. Mark Hyman

The history of human civilization on nearly every continent shows that humankind has created its own pharmacy over thousands of years of experimentation and observation of nature and has used it in times of weakness or illness. Traditional Eastern medicine is known for this approach and is perhaps the only medicine to have treated people for centuries by concentrating on four human aspects, i.e., our bodily, psychological, spiritual, and cosmic dimensions.

Practitioners use herbs, essential oils, bee products, and even precious stones and minerals. Medications have been known to people for ages. Yet, synthetic drugs, compared with our evolutionary time frame, are a completely new, unnatural phenomenon: humans are attempting to defeat disease by introducing artificial substances into a living organism.

It is important to be cognizant of the fact that this means introducing *something foreign* from the outside world to your natural inner world. When this process occurs, your body must first recognize the delivery of such a material and take it apart into substances it knows, not losing but gaining energy in the process. These foreign, external substances—synthetic drugs—introduce chaos and disrupt your body's inner balance.

Your cellular receptors and enzymes are blocked. Your entire biological structure is poisoned. Energy that is necessary for life is directed toward detoxifying your embattled body.

I am deeply convinced the body has a natural potential for self-repair. It has sufficient inner healing power to return its disrupted functioning to a state of harmony and balance. Such a position absolutely does not exclude taking advantage of the achievements of modern medicine and does not dispute the obvious need for medical facilities and the work of physicians.

Quite the contrary, I have the utmost respect and esteem for the knowledgeable representatives of each field of life and science who are open to new knowledge and experiments. I follow the current achievements of medicine with admiration and am fascinated by their courageous goals. We are extremely fortunate that, as we progress through the twenty-first century, those medical specialists will achieve even more improvements to this realm where what was once impossible becomes possible.

However, I will do everything in my power to use medical achievements (like synthetic drugs or bypass for example) only in cases where it is absolutely necessary.

As the old saying goes, the road to hell is paved with good intentions. I'm not against conventional medicine. I believe that in certain cases, it's necessary to entrust your health to your doctors, to take the medications they order, and to follow the treatment they prescribe. I don't exclude that possibility at all. I argue, however, that we should make a greater effort to maintain our health as a preventative measure, to improve our quality of life, and to take care of our own bodies. According to the ancient Ayurvedic proverb, *If your diet is wrong, medicine is of no use. If your diet is correct, medicine is of no need.*

When we give our body the right amount of sleep, good food, movement, and recreation, it can repay us with good health and a reliable physical condition. Our joy in existence and the possibility of complete spiritual and intellectual growth follows naturally from that.

Controversies Surrounding Medications

In addition to real illnesses, we can also count
many others which are only imagined, for which
physicians have invented imaginary medications.
These ailments go by many names, just like
the medicines that are made for them.
—Jonathan Swift

At the turn of the twenty-first century, it became widely believed that the pharmaceutical industry could deliver magical products that would easily and quickly solve all our health problems. People have thus been freed of all responsibility for their health. After all, the right medicine is enough to get rid of troublesome infections and to allow you to forget about your suffering.

The ancient Greeks used the term *pharmakon* to designate not only medicine (herbal medicine) but also poison. We often forget this double-sided nature of medication, administering it in good faith to ourselves and others, often to the point of absurdity.

The United States (among many other countries) suffers from a serious drug addiction problem, which can be traced back to painkiller overprescription. These days, according to the US surgeon general, more Americans use prescription opioids than smoke cigarettes.[229] More Americans are killed by opiates like oxycodone, hydrocodone, fentanyl, and morphine than by car accidents.[230] According to the surgeon general's report, twenty-seven million Americans took opioids at some point in 2015. Comedian John Oliver turned a critical eye on the growing drug epidemic in October 2016,[231] noting that the problem's origins lie in narcotic painkillers and the drug companies that falsely denied their addictive nature, recommending them as safe for different kinds of pain. We know better now, so it's crucial that you keep in mind these drugs' addictive qualities and seriously consider your need for them.

Each of us has heard many times when we have complained of a headache, "Why suffer? Take a pill and you'll be fine!" It's easier that way! However, there are many ailments whose causes haven't been explained by the research. This includes

---

[229] Dr. Mercola, "Opioid Addiction Now Surpasses Smoking," Mercola.com, last modified November 29, 2016, http://articles.mercola.com/sites/articles/archive/2016/11/29/opioid-addiction-surpasses-smoking.aspx?#_edn1.

[230] Ibid.

[231] Ibid.

certain types of headaches. Pain is one of the most important signals of illness, its key symptom. Muffling it with a pill can cause us to ignore or miss a more serious condition that, if ignored, could lead to tragedy.

In general, medications don't remove the root cause but simply quiet the symptoms of the disease by blocking certain types of chemical reactions in the body. They work by connecting to cellular receptors: natural hooks that chemical substances, such as hormones, latch on to and that trigger many types of reactions. The problem is they also connect to unrelated receptors. These additional processes result in serious problems, the so-called side effects and adverse reactions that we all know from those patient information inserts.

Let's look at the generally available information on statins—lipid-lowering medications that reduce cardiovascular disease and mortality in those who are at high risk. Statins, unfortunately, can also cause a series of serious side effects. For example, they block the production and inflow of coenzyme Q10 (CoQ10) to mitochondria, where internal cellular energy conversion takes place. CoQ10 is a natural antioxidant that helps our body fight free radicals: atoms or molecules that contain unpaired electrons, which intercept (steal) the electrons of healthy cells and are the cause of the cells' degeneration, i.e., aging, weakness, illness, and death.

Interrupting the mitochondria's work weakens our body's ability to produce energy. A person experiences this as constant fatigue and has the feeling that he or she could fall asleep on his or her feet. Other side effects also include pain in the fingers and toes and unpleasant knee ailments, which doctors often interpret as rheumatic pain. One large Finnish study found that people taking statins had an almost 50 percent higher risk of developing type 2 diabetes. According to the report, statins appear to increase the risk of type 2 diabetes by increasing a person's insulin resistance and impairing the pancreas's ability to secrete insulin.[232]

So, we can see that all pharmaceuticals have their pros and cons. The former are emphasized in advertisements, while the producer has a legal obligation to inform users of the latter in attached informational leaflets. This results in an insert written in painfully small, distracting print, using numerous specialized terms the average consumer has a hard time understanding.

Frequent colds during spring, fall, or a mild winter are caused by over two hundred different viruses. We all know the symptoms: sore throat, fever, chills, cough, fatigue, sullen mood, watery eyes, and a stuffy nose, which usually appear a few days after infection.

There are those who get a flu shot each year in order to build up their body's immunity. Let's remember, however, that this method only provides temporary immunity. Some of us decide to take antibiotics, ignoring the fact that they only kill bacteria and not viruses, which are the true cause of the cold. Surely nobody will give up cough syrup. Let's take a look then at a typical cough syrup, which we've bought over the counter and which we plan to use several times a day.

We usually don't know and thus don't consider that such treatment hampers and even obviates the work of our natural

---

[232] Dennis Thompson, "Statins Linked to Raised Risk of Type 2 Diabetes," *HealthDay News*, accessed June 2, 2017, http://www.webmd.com/diabetes/news/20150304/statins-linked-to-raised-risk-of-type-2-diabetes#1.

immune system. Taking cough syrup every few hours for a few days can significantly prolong the time necessary for a complete recovery.

This happens because we lower our fever, which is our main defense against viruses; we block the production of mucus, which is meant to flush the viruses to our stomach so that hydrochloric acid can deal with them; and we needlessly dry out our sinuses to breathe better. This actually causes them to swell, which makes it harder to get air through the nose, and so we open our mouths to get some air into our lungs. This, in turn, leaves our throat completely defenseless.

By muffling our cough and fighting the unpleasant symptoms of a cold, we stifle our loyal and devoted defense mechanisms, while not actually eliminating the real culprits! All the symptoms of a cold are, in fact, our best and most effective army protecting us against an enemy invasion, and we, like saboteurs, interfere with its performance of duties it has known for millions of years, which were created by evolution. Remember, coughing is a good thing. It is how we eliminate secretions, irritants, and nasty microbes that our bodies would prefer to do without. This natural response helps to protect us from illness and potentially harmful toxins in the environment. *The human body is truly remarkable!*

In contrast, I will quote here the words of Dr. Daniel Kalish (*Your Guide to Healthy Hormones*), so you can better understand these examples and the goal of this part of our discussion:

> From my perspective, people should get healthier
> as they get older. In fact, my healthiest female

patients are what I call my *over-80 club*. They provide living proof that you can get healthier as you age. These folks, all in their 80s, are sexually active, use no medications, exercise daily, and are emotionally vital and mentally sharp. They share certain lifelong traits: they are long-term exercise fanatics, follow good diets, have had rich and satisfying personal relationships, and are intellectually engaged in stimulating mental activities.

Remember

- Our body and soul are priceless sources of information about ourselves; let's learn to interpret the signals they send in times of crisis.
- Pain is a perfect, well-formed, and sensitive alarm system that nature has equipped human and animal organisms with.
- The state of human health has been a challenge for doctors and scientists for thousands of years, but it is the most important task for each of us as well.
- Health is nothing more than taking responsibility for ourselves.
- The right lifestyle is a better guarantee of health than pharmaceutical supplements.

CHAPTER 16

FROM THE SACRED TO THE PROFANE, OR A FEW WORDS ON SALT

There must be something sacred in salt.
It is in our tears and in the ocean.
—Khalil Gibran

Known to every society on every continent for thousands of years, salt is a substance that makes good health and tasty food possible. Throughout the ages, salt was prized for its preservative properties, since the compound itself never goes bad and it prevents any organic material from spoiling.

Salt has also played a role in various religious circles in many cultures, forming an ever-present element of all sorts of offerings to the gods and magical substances—without it, their effectiveness would be difficult to imagine. Sorcery, witchcraft, incantations, oaths, and even wars, financial settlements, and friendships have had to take salt's presence into account.

Ancient wanderers, coming across long-stagnant water, would decontaminate it using lumps of salt. This custom is even seen in the Bible, when Elishah helped save the lives and health of the people around him. He went out to the spring, threw the salt into it, and healed the water so that no more unfruitfulness would come from it.

Salt was and still is not only a common seasoning, preservative, and disinfectant but also a multilayered symbol tied to numerous customs and superstitions, all of them testaments to the respect in which it is held. In his *Natural History*, over two thousand years ago, Pliny the Elder devoted numerous remarks to salt and considered bread and salt to be praiseworthy features of a simple, healthy, and natural lifestyle. He admired this phenomenal substance for the way it "keeps a person of sound mind throughout his life, and after death delays the decomposition of the body for a long time, thus fulfilling the role played by the soul during life."

He believed, "There are two things of utmost importance in the world: sun and salt." Salt's exceptional status and the great desire for it can be seen in the ancient Roman practice of the *salarium*, or "salt-money"—a special sum for purchasing lumps of salt, so that nobody would have to go without.

For many reasons, salt was an expensive yet essential product. The owners of salt mines and salt works ranked among any society's wealthiest. They became rich remarkably quickly, ensuring great fortunes for themselves and their descendants. Salt was also used during important life and business events.

In Arab culture, it remains a sign of hospitality, friendship, loyalty, and lasting interpersonal relationships to this day. In ancient Israel, contracts were finalized, oaths sworn, true friendships sealed, and promises of marriage bound by both sides eating a few grains of salt.

Observing how salt could be obtained by evaporating sea water led to the concept of salt as a gift from the gods, sent down to support human health, riches, wisdom, vitality, and—above all—life. It was also noted that, by some incomprehensible magic, salt also existed within us, as revealed by the taste of our blood, sweat, and tears. A salt oath was especially powerful and considered sacred in ancient times.

This special human attitude toward salt arose from the way its properties were used, experience of the results, and observation of the processes in which it took part. So, how did salt become known as the "white death" in the latter half of the twentieth century and how was this timeless superstar thrown from its pedestal with a bang? What caused this paragon's fall from grace?

Today, nobody needs convincing of salt's profound significance to our health. In its natural form, both sea salt and mined salt are a true treasure trove of macro- and microelements, such as potassium, magnesium, sodium, calcium, iodine, lithium, selenium, zinc, copper, chromium, iron, and manganese. Food tastes better and is also much more nutritious thanks to salt. Humans' and some animals' natural craving for salt is not a cruel joke by some capricious Creator but a clear biological mechanism prompting us to supply our bodies with this "substance of life."

It is easy to see how wisely evolution has equipped us and our animal brethren with this inner drive to consume salt. Every dog owner has observed how eagerly his or her pet licks salty, sweaty hands. Cattle breeders and foresters give their animals "salt licks," large blocks of rock salt that serve as an excellent supplement to these four-legged creatures' diet.

We should remember that the salt in sea water formed part of the natural environment in which our genetic code bathed itself for billions of years, later to morph into numerous forms and shape the human body. So, we can see that consuming salt and its presence in the human corpus are closely entwined in a synergistic network of many different elements and processes, precisely woven by the astonishingly logical and effective course of evolution.

Without salt, countless biochemical reactions in the human body would be impossible. Enzyme activity and energy and hormone production, as well as the transporting of protein, would be disrupted, threatening the state of our entire system.

The saline concentration in human blood must be kept constant. The daily salt requirement for healthy adults is five to fifteen grams. This is not a fixed amount, since physical effort, heat, illnesses that increase sweating, and our diet can all lead to an increased need for salt. Human sweat is about 0.5 percent salt.

If we don't supply our bodies with enough salt, our endocrine system compensates by limiting the amount of salt excreted in our sweat and urine. On a restrictive, salt-free diet, the body gradually loses small amounts of salt via the urinary system and sweat glands. If strenuous physical activity is added to this uncomfortable mix, the saline loss intensifies. The human corpus tries to protect itself by releasing more water, so that the right level of salt in the blood is maintained. The result of these necessary defense mechanisms is progressive dehydration and in the end, death. We die of thirst!

Many dietary topics become argumentative playing fields, where endless debates roil among experts lobbing concrete arguments and research back and forth. The controversy surrounding salt is no exception to these scientific skirmishes. Such moments may recall the words of Ray Bradbury (of *Fahrenheit 451* fame): "One professor calling another an idiot, one philosopher screaming down another's gullet. All of them running about, putting out the stars and extinguishing the sun."

It's worth looking at some opinions from the not-too-distant past, as well as those currently in the media. The last few years of the twentieth century were full of loud appeals by dieticians to limit our salt intake, since the research indicated a link between salt consumption and high blood pressure. The latest findings of many research centers have revealed this to be false, and scientists now say that limiting our salt intake can do more harm than good.

Salt is responsible for regulating blood volume and pressure, as well as maintaining the elasticity of our blood vessels. Our blood pressure can be affected by many things: stress, age, level of physical activity, genetic predispositions, and diet. Some people who are particularly sensitive to salt, and specifically the sodium in salt, may experience elevated blood pressure in reaction to salt consumption, but most of this rise is due to completely different causes.

I've already mentioned how all traditional populations used salt in their cuisine. This observation includes peoples who settled far from the sea and salt mines and who did not import it from other regions. How did they manage? By burning salt-rich plants, they obtained a special ash that could be added like a spice to the dishes they made.

Salt consists of two crucial elements for our health and lives: sodium and chloride ions, which our bodies are unable to produce on their own. They must be supplied through a proper diet. Sodium is a bioelement that plays a key role in the human body's physiology. It helps maintain the right concentration of acids and bases. Around 40 percent of this mineral is found in our bones, 5 percent in our organs and cells, and 55 percent in our blood plasma and extracellular fluid. It affects the condition of our nervous system, supports the transport of various nutrients to our cells, and regulates blood pressure.

Chloride ions, meanwhile, regulate the volume and pressure of our blood and the pH of our bodily fluids. They play a key role in maintaining acid-base balance, muscle activity, fluid movement throughout the body, hydrochloric acid production, and the proper functioning of our brain and nervous system. While sodium is present in many different foods, chloride ions are not. They must be obtained from salt. They participate in carbohydrate digestion by activating the enzyme amylase.

Our saline needs are highly individualized and differ from person to person. People with weak adrenal glands lose greater amounts of salt in their urine, so they must consume more. Others, meanwhile, must limit the salt in their diet; otherwise, they risk calcium loss in their bones, which could cause osteoporosis, and potassium loss in the body. Too little salt in the food we eat leads to a weakened sense of taste, chronic fatigue, difficulty breathing during exercise, general weakness, and muscle cramps in the fingers and calves.

Dr. Edward Howell, mentioned earlier, noted that populations that follow a primarily raw diet (e.g., the Inuit) do not need to add too much salt to their food. Consumers of industrially processed and cooked foods, however, should add salt as a necessity, since salt activates the digestive enzymes in the intestines. Eating salted food is thus beneficial in every respect.

Inhabitants of regions where sea salt is used know this well. Such salt is not refined and thus not deprived of its most valuable nutrients, which in most places are thrown carelessly away along with the mother liquor following the crystallization process. This extremely harmful procedure is carried out on mined salt and sea salt, which are changed into bleached, pure sodium chloride, stripped of all its macro- and microelements.

Most of the debate on this topic avoids the problem of refined, purified salt, also known as kitchen or table salt. Many of us, standing in front of the salt display at the store, choose one that looks neat and tidy, is bright white, and pours easily. Manufacturers know our weaknesses well and pour their purified salt into transparent packaging. Let's not give in to these clever marketing tricks!

Few of us know that such salt, like sugar, flour, and vegetable oils, is highly refined. The result is a chemical product that, processed at high temperatures, has completely lost most of its precious minerals, including its essential magnesium.

To make sure the salt is dry and loose, producers of this "perfect" product mercilessly stuff it full of harmful additives, including aluminum. Modern technology also removes its natural iodide in the process, only to replace it later with potassium iodide at levels that can be toxic to our bodies.[233] To stabilize the volatile iodide compound, they add dextrose, which turns the iodized salt purple. The white color demanded by consumers is achieved by using numerous bleaching agents.

The presence of salt in our diet is no trend or novelty but a continuation of one of the human body's most ancient natural needs. Salt is vital to us, and we can't function in good health or develop properly without it. But the table salt offered by producers and the salt found in every processed food, including bread, is not the salt that our bodies really need.

Such salt has nothing in common with its natural counterpart. Instead, it is a highly toxic product that must be dealt with by our livers. However, the liver is only able to neutralize about four grams of this salt daily; after all, it's got other toxins to process from the industrially processed foods we consume.

Industrially refined natural salt (sea salt or mined) is 98 percent sodium chloride (NaCl) along with artificial chemical substances.[234] These include chemical compounds that absorb moisture, as well as ferrocyanide and aluminosilicate. Some countries where the water is not fluoridated also add fluoride to their table salt. In France, 35 percent of the salt offered for sale contains either sodium fluoride or potassium fluoride. Fluoridated salt is quite widespread in South America.

[233] Mary Enig, *Eat Fat Lose Fat*, 96.
[234] Mercola, "Add Salt to Your Food Daily—Despite What Your Doctor Says," accessed April 22, 2015, https://articles.mercola.com/sites/articles/archive/2011/09/20/salt-myth.aspx.

Salt's presence in so many foods tempts health officials on every continent to enrich it with substances meant to stop certain plagues of civilization, such as tooth decay, thyroid conditions, improper bone structure, and so on. Recently, salt has begun to be enriched with folic acid, and some countries also plan to add iron.

The term "sea salt" was long associated only with a healthy, natural substance but has since been adopted by clever producers and retailers, who place it on packages of sea salt produced using industrial methods! The best, healthiest salt is that which is obtained from sea water dried by the sun in huge, clay-lined vats. It is known as *fire from water*, since it harnesses the amazing power of the two elements of fire and water—or, in this case, sun and water.

This salt contains traces of sea life, which delivers natural iodine and calcium. Its light-gray color indicates it has a high moisture content and contains many bioelements. The aesthetically inclined among us shouldn't be scared off by this alleged *dirt*; such "contamination" should encourage everyone to use this natural treasure that our bodies need so badly. It may be hard to believe, but such salt consists of 82 percent sodium chloride, 14 percent macroelements (mainly magnesium), and eighty other trace minerals![235]

A lack of salt in our diet manifests in the human body in many ways. The clearest signs are strong thirst, fatigue, drowsiness, loss of appetite, nausea, vomiting, and difficulty concentrating. We lose significant amounts of salt during heat waves and vigorous physical activity, but also when we

---

[235] Mary Enig, *Eat Fat Lose Fat*, 96.

experience bleeding, diarrhea, or heavy menstruation. In such situations, we need to increase the salt in our daily diet.

Considering all the aspects of salt discussed here, I recommend consuming unrefined, natural salt. I particularly recommend Celtic[236] salt and Himalayan sea salt. Once you've taken an interest in these ecological treasures, I suggest you also check out unrefined French and New Zealand salt, since they aren't contaminated with mercury or heavy metals like salts from other maritime regions.

Although I continue to stress the true benefits of unprocessed natural salt, this doesn't mean that we can consume it in uncontrolled, unlimited amounts. According to Morton Satin, PhD, the vice president of science and research at the Salt Institute, "the fundamental indicator of salt intake sufficiency points to 1.5 teaspoons (8 grams) of salt per day as the basic human requirement."[237] Here, we still need to exercise moderation! For many of the biochemical processes in our bodies to run properly, finding the right proportion of sodium to potassium is of utmost importance. Upsetting this ratio could lead to high blood pressure, memory loss, improper muscle contractions, disruption of heart functioning and nerve impulse transmission, erectile dysfunction, and many other issues.

The simplest way to avoid these problems is to give up processed food, which has a consistently low level of potassium along with a high level of sodium. Proper cellular and tissue function and many of the physiological processes in our

---

236   The Celtic word for salt meant "holy" or "sacred."

237   Morton Satin, "Exposing Mainstream Myths," accessed May 29, 2018, https://www.westonaprice.org/health-topics/abcs-of-nutrition/salt-and-our-health/.

bodies depend upon numerous mineral components provided by a sensible diet.

Even a basic understanding of the mechanisms of our metabolism and the energy in our bodies can allow us to identify our dietary needs for elements that will later serve as building blocks, energy sources, and regulating substances. Then, we can decide what kind of diet we want, what it should consist of, how much food to eat, and the factors ensuring its proper digestion, absorption, and use.

I will continue to repeat this one simple conclusion: we should eat unprocessed food from organic farms and breeders to ensure the optimal supply of the natural nutrients that support our health and proper functioning. Unrefined, natural sea salt or mined salt should be added to our list of essential, nutritious, and truly organic foods.

I should add a few more sentences here in support of these final conclusions. However, I'll just seal my discussion with the words "I swear on salt," since the phrase was a highly trusted and esteemed assurance in ancient times.

In conclusion, I will just add two more thoughts, each of them beginning with the word *apparently*. Apparently, all negative powers, demons, wicked witches, and curses lose their terrible, destructive power in the face of salt. Since the Middle Ages, salt has been believed to ward off bad omens. It is added to holy water in some Christian traditions to this day.

Apparently, spilling salt is not only a great loss but also a sign of imminent bad luck, trouble, strife, worry, and destruction. One sign of this belief is Leonardo da Vinci's placement of an overturned saltcellar before the figure of Judas in his famous *Last Supper*.

So, it's important to have salt handy, not only for health and culinary reasons. Making sure it doesn't spill, of course, may reflect an appreciation for tidiness and a desire to save money, but it also shows respect for salt's exceptional and diverse assets, among which even these more questionable ones may prove important.

Remember

- Bleached, refined salt that has been deprived of its micro- and macroelements is incredibly harmful.
- Eliminating industrially refined salt (pure NaCl) and replacing it with its original form is sure to have a healthy impact.
- Salting our dishes comes from a natural need to provide our bodies with bioelements that are essential to our health and lives.
- Our need for salt is quite individual and depends on many factors (physical activity, heat, fever, and so on).
- Strong thirst is the first crucial sign of a lack of salt in our diet.
- Too little salt in our diet is quite damaging to the human corpus and can seriously hinder its proper functioning and development.
- Salt is not only a popular seasoning but also a source of many other components that are essential to nearly all the biochemical processes taking place in the body.

CHAPTER 17

IN SEARCH OF NECTAR

What is alive lives on moisture, and what is
dead dries up; the seeds of all things are moist
and all nourishment contains juice.
—Greek philosopher

Every form of life on earth is tied to the primeval ocean in which it existed four billion years ago and where it developed exclusively until the end of the Cambrian Period (ca. 500 million years ago). Oceans and seas cover around 71 percent of the earth's surface.[238] A wealth of processes taking place on our planet over millions of years led to the creation of countless living organisms whose lives are inextricably connected with water.

Water is a fundamental component of the tissue structure of living organisms, including humans, both in terms of sheer amount and biochemical importance. Human muscles are around 80 percent water, while the blood is around 85 percent, human bones nearly 45 percent, and the brain around 80 percent. A constant, sufficient level of water in the human body is necessary for it to function and stay alive. A loss of

---

[238] *Wielki ilustrowany atlas świata* [Large Illustrated Atlas of the World], 184.

around 10 percent of our body water is considered unsafe for our health, while 20 percent is considered life-threatening and usually leads to death.[239]

The amount of water in the human body must be continually replenished, since it is expelled in the urine, feces, sweat, and exhalation from the lungs. This water level is determined not only by our diet but also the temperature of our environment, our level of physical activity, and our overall condition.

At high temperatures and under intense sunlight, the human body can survive only two to three days without water, while in more moderate climes, we can last from a week to ten to twelve days. In extreme conditions and during strenuous physical activity, a healthy adult can lose as much as ten liters (approximately 2.5 gallons) of water. This shortage is signaled by intense thirst, dry mucous membranes, weakness, headache, and even loss of consciousness.

Our water levels can be replenished by consuming various beverages. The global market offers so many different kinds it's hard to know which ones are suitable and healthy for us. This is especially true since the labels of nearly all such drinks assure us they contain vitamins, mineral salts, microelements, natural fruit and vegetable juices, water from the oldest and deepest layers of the earth, and so on. However, we already know we should be wary of such assurances by producers and proceed with caution.

[239] Chlebińska, *Anatomia i fizjologia człowieka* [Human Anatomy and Physiology] (Warsaw: Wydawnictwa Szkolne i Pedagogiczne, 1975), 287.

Soda

Dieticians warn that the main contributing factor to the plague of degenerative diseases now tormenting our civilized world is global society's weakness for carbonated and sweetened drinks like cola, sodas, and so on. The average American drinks around 216 liters (approximately 54 US gallons) of such beverages a year, while around 130 billion liters (approximately 32.5 billion US gallons) of cola are consumed annually worldwide.[240]

Decades of extensive advertising campaigns and clever product placement in TV shows and films have made these beverages ubiquitous. They've even found their way into the hands of consumers who were long shielded from such harmful products: children. Today, these beverages are for sale in every school snack shop or hallway vending machine. New generations are growing up recklessly guzzling gallons of soda with no concern for the consequences. This is yet another argument to take care of yourself, since the chances are slim that our obese children, poisoned by these drinks, will be able to help give us a dignified life in our old age! A single can of cola or similar beverage contains around ten teaspoons of sugar! This is shocking not only because of the amount but also the quality of the sugar. That sugar is fructose, obtained from the worst product we know (which I've written about earlier): corn syrup.

---

[240] "Countries Compared by Lifestyle > Food and Drink > Soft Drink > Consumption," International Statistics at NationMaster.com, Global Market Information Database, published by Euromonitor. Aggregates compiled by Nation Master," accessed 2002, http://www.nationmaster.com/country-info/stats/Lifestyle/Food-and-drink/Soft-drink/Consumption.

There are some consumers who try to "take care of themselves" and opt for "light" versions of these drinks. They think they're making the right choice by avoiding harmful sugar, but they're really jumping out of the frying pan and into the fire. These beverages are full of artificial sweeteners like aspartame.

Such sugar substitutes are much more harmful than sugar and just as addictive. The most common one is aspartame, which is often hidden behind the symbol E951. Sugar substitutes can cause many health problems, the most common of which include dizziness, impaired vision, intense muscle pain, numbness in the limbs, pancreatitis, high blood pressure, retinal hemorrhage, tremors, and depression. Aspartame is suspected of causing birth defects and chemical imbalances in the brain. It is poison!

Aspartame can be found in thousands of other products as well, from chewing gum to vitamin supplements and toothpaste. Researchers at Utah State University have shown that even small doses of this substance can cause adverse changes in the pituitary glands of mice.[241] All the biochemical processes in the human body depend on this gland to run properly.

Incidentally, aspartame was discovered by mistake. In 1965, chemist James M. Schlatter was trying to develop a drug for peptic ulcer disease. Once day, he accidentally spilled one of the chemicals he was using onto his finger. Probably

---

[241] Jim Earles, *Sugar-Free Blues: Everything You Wanted to Know about Artificial Sweeteners*, accessed June 23, 2018, https://www.westonaprice.org/health-topics/modern-foods/sugar-free-blues-everything-you-wanted-to-know-about-artificial-sweeteners/#aspartame.

violating a million lab safety standards, he proceeded to lick his finger, noting the chemical's sweet taste—and thus one of the most dangerous and controversial food additives in history was born.[242]

Dr. H. J. Roberts, author of *Aspartame Disease: An Ignored Epidemic* and an expert in the field, states clearly in one documentary, "Aspartame is not a food but is, in fact, a poison." When digested, aspartame is broken down into the amino acids phenylalanine and aspartic acid, as well as methanol. This last component is widely known as a dangerous toxin.

It can also be found in small amounts in fruit juices. In response, producers claim that methanol isn't as dangerous as scientists would have us believe. They ignore the fact that carbonated beverages contain fifteen to one hundred times more methanol than fruit juices. Either way, a safe concentration of methanol has yet to be determined.

In addition to sugar or sweeteners, most drinks also contain phosphoric acid. One sign of it is an audible "pop" when you open your drink. This acid blocks magnesium and calcium absorption, which can lead to broken bones in children at their first substantial fall.

Most of these drinks also contain caffeine. Both caffeine and theobromine (in tea and cocoa) behave like sugar in our bodies. Within a mere forty minutes of consuming these substances, your blood pressure rises, your adrenal glands are activated, your adrenaline production increases, and your blood sugar climbs.

---

[242] Dr. Mercola, "Artificial Sweeteners—More Dangerous than You Ever Imagined," Mercola.com, last updated October 13, 2009, http://articles.mercola.com/sites/articles/archive/2009/10/13/artificial-sweeteners-more-dangerous-than-you-ever-imagined.aspx.

An hour after these symptoms occur, the human body feels tired and requires another dose of stimulants. This is a vicious cycle leading to addiction and numerous health problems.

Sugar increases your insulin levels, leads to excessive weight gain, raises your blood pressure and bad cholesterol, and causes heart disease, diabetes, and premature aging as well as many other negative side effects. It is just as addictive as any narcotic and wreaks havoc in the human body. Caffeine also irritates the stomach mucosa, upsetting the organ's acid balance.

In addition to the substances I've just presented, most beverage producers "improve" their goods with other additives: artificial dyes, flavors, preservatives, and flavor enhancers.

We shouldn't let ourselves be taken in by the lovely, intense fruit or vegetable aromas of many drinks. These aromas are made in chemical laboratories. The fragrance of fresh pears is really ethyl acetate and that of pineapples is ethyl butyrate, while butyl acetate gives us the scent of bananas. There are countless other examples, since the food industry has mastered these esters. These compounds are present in nature and do their job well (e.g., attracting insects), but most drinks do not contain these chemicals in a form that Mother Nature created. People who want to take care of their bodies and care about their health and loved ones should never drink such beverages. They should be eliminated from our diets once and for all!

Coffee

Most of us know the pleasant, refined aroma of this next drink, which is consumed with delight not only in the morning but also in many other situations. And although it is an addictive drug, almost nobody feels any guilt over downing several cups a day. It is easy to guess the protagonist of our discussion: natural coffee, for centuries the most popular beverage in the world next to water.

Although it only appeared in Europe in the sixteenth century, coffee was already known by the first millennium BCE, in what is now Ethiopia. The natives harvested the ripe berries of the coffee plants growing there to then eat them cooked with a bit of fat. They were prized for their energizing, refreshing properties and their ability to ward off exhaustion and fatigue, as well as stimulate the mind. The berries were believed to deliver a burst of energy to travelers, hunters, and warriors. They were also ascribed magical powers, since they fought off sleep, increased alertness, and guaranteed the vigilance of guards and shepherds.

The Bedouins spread coffee throughout Arabia, adopting the custom of roasting, grinding, and brewing the beans from Arab merchants traveling on trade throughout Yemen. Islam was long hostile to the drink, and its consumption was officially prohibited in Mecca in 1511. However, because of its exceptional popularity, the ban was soon lifted. A German botanist traveling through Africa in the latter half of the sixteenth century noted that "a beverage black as ink" was consumed by the natives "in the morning, in open areas and without the slightest hint of fear or caution."[243]

Several centuries have passed since those observations were made, and today around seven million tons of coffee are

---

[243] "Odkrycie kawy" [Discovering Coffee], http://sirius.cs.put.poznan.pl/~inf89810/html/historia.html.

produced in various regions of the world (Brazil, Vietnam, Columbia, Indonesia, India, Ethiopia, Peru, Mexico, Guatemala, and Honduras), with nearly five hundred billion cups downed each year.

Coffee is available in many forms: as raw, unroasted beans ("green" coffee), roasted, instant, ground, flavored, and decaf. Its price depends on many factors; since the twentieth century, it has not been exorbitantly high, although kopi luwak, the most expensive variety, costs around thirty dollars per cup.

This coffee is obtained from beans that have been eaten by an animal known as the luwak, or Asian palm civet, pushed through its digestive tract, and then collected from the animal's feces and washed, roasted, and ground. The beans then make their way from Indonesia into the cups of coffee connoisseurs around the world, particularly in Japan, the United States, and China.

Some African communities gathered coffee beans to form chewable balls by mixing the crushed beans with fat. These were chewed on long journeys, during strenuous physical activity, before a visit to one's beloved, or during battle. After all, they were believed to provide strength, fight off sleep, reduce physical and psychological fatigue, and increase sexual desire.

Do contemporary studies of coffee confirm these opinions? There is a wealth of conflicting conclusions on the world's most popular beverage. Some praise its benefits, while others warn against the damage it can cause to our health. For example, one of the benefits of coffee, when it's consumed in moderation, is helping to lower the risk of Alzheimer's disease. Dr. Arfran Ikram, an assistant professor in neuroepidemiology at Erasmus Medical Centre Rotterdam, believes that the polyphenol and caffeine helps to reduce inflammation and deterioration of brain cells in the areas of the brain involved in memory.[244]

From another point of view, maintaining a constant blood sugar level by cutting down on potentially disruptive products should be a healthy habit for all of us. Does coffee also contribute to such harmful blood sugar fluctuations? Dr. Walter C. Willett from the Harvard School of Public Health states that "coffee is an unusually strong collection of biologically active compounds."[245] Like any food, it has far-reaching effects on our bodies, and it should be treated like a powerful drug.

Caffeine only makes up about 1 to 2 percent of coffee beans' content. Yet it is the component whose impact on the human body has been most studied by scientists and is universally applied in medicine. The remaining substances, such as chlorogenic acid, caffeol, polyphenols, phytoestrogens, and diterpenes, are still within researchers' field of interest.

Of course, this doesn't mean that coffee is the devil's work and should be absolutely forbidden—as was the case for Christians until the time of Pope Clemens VIII, who revoked the ban and freed the custom of coffee drinking from the realm of sinful secrecy.

However, despite these conflicting opinions, there are still eight reasons to consider giving up coffee:

[244] *Coffee Buying Guide*, accessed May 29, 2018, https://www.foodmatters.com/coffee-buying-guide.

[245] R. M. Van Dam, W. C. Willett, J. E. Manson, and F. B. Hu, "Coffee, Caffeine, and Risk of Type 2 Diabetes: A Prospective Cohort Study in Younger and Middle-Aged US Women," *Diabetes Care* 2 (2006): 398–403.

1. The caffeine in coffee raises stress hormone levels in the body. Higher concentrations of these hormones in the blood powerfully stimulate the organs and various tissues, thus excessively exploiting them. This leads to fatigue and diminished well-being.
2. A caffeine habit reduces our sensitivity to insulin, making it harder for the body to react to unstable blood sugar levels.
3. Unfiltered coffee does have the highest antioxidant content, but when we drink it, significant amounts of diterpenes also enter our bodies, causing an increase in triglycerides, LDL cholesterol, and VLDL cholesterol.[246]
4. The chlorogenic acids in coffee, which may delay glucose absorption in the intestines, also increase homocysteine levels[247]—a risk factor for cardiovascular disease.
5. Coffee's acidity is tied to gastrointestinal discomfort, indigestion, heartburn, and imbalanced intestinal flora. It provides an excellent fuel for the growth of harmful bacteria in the gut.
6. Coffee addiction is a serious problem for its consumers. It prevents them from choosing natural and healthy

[246] Axel F. Sigurdsson, "Benefits of Coffee—Caffeine Benefits Explained," accessed May 29, 2018, https://www.docsopinion.com/2015/03/12/health-benefits-of-coffee-the-scientific-evidence/.

[247] "Consumption of high doses of chlorogenic acid, present in coffee, or of black tea increases plasma total homocysteine concentrations in humans," *American Journal of Clinical Nutrition* 73, no. 3, (March 2001): 532–538, https://doi.org/10.1093/ajcn/73.3.532, accessed May 24, 2018, via https://academic.oup.com/ajcn/article/73/3/532/4737354.

sources of energy for their bodies. Coming off coffee is a very difficult time for addicts, and they feel truly awful! I speak from my own experience.

7. 5-HIAA is an organic acid that is also one of the components of serotonin. Coffee-lovers have increased levels of this acid in their urine, meaning that it has been flushed from the body and is no longer present to participate in its typical processes in the brain. The result is low serotonin, nervousness, disrupted sleep, mood swings, unstable energy levels, and intestinal dysfunction.

Yet another vicious cycle emerges: a person who is tired, irritated, and sensitive and had a bad night's sleep will reach for another cup of coffee to get back on his or her feet. This is the caffeine-related anxiety so well-known to doctors, which is a result of excess coffee consumption. I would just add that a dose of 1,000 milligrams of caffeine a day, or around eight cups of coffee, is highly toxic to the human body, although the minimum lethal dose is thought to be three times that amount.

In seventeenth-century England, coffee was sold only in pharmacies because of common overdoses among coffee lovers, who treated coffee like a panacea for many illnesses and ailments (including alcoholism). Until the end of the nineteenth century, noble estates and wealthy burgher homes in Poland employed *kawiarki*—specialists who would not only oversee the roasting, grinding, and brewing of the beans but would also purchase the right coffee and make sure that every member of the household or guests received the correct number of cups.

Coffee was served exclusively in porcelain cups, as it was believed that such dishes protected people from being poisoned. Later, faience became an acceptable alternative to porcelain.

8. Frequent, heavy urination is another reason that coffee drinking is detrimental. This phenomenon causes important minerals, such as calcium, magnesium, and potassium to be flushed from the body in greater amounts. Disrupting our electrolyte balance can lead to serious health complications throughout the body.

Anyone who is feeling out of sorts, tired, and absentminded and is experiencing symptoms of chronic stress should consider cutting down coffee consumption to the minimum—one cup a day. Anyone with any sort of infection or hormonal or emotional problems should do the same.

I encourage you to perform an interesting and useful experiment on yourself. It should last for about a month, to make sure your observations and conclusions are reliable. During this time, eliminate all forms of coffee and observe how you feel and function. I'll give you a few tried-and-true ways to do so, but I will stress that those who previously consumed relatively large amounts of caffeine, alcohol, or sugar as well as those with the greatest toxin levels can have the hardest time in the beginning. Physical symptoms, such as headache, tiredness, drowsiness, and fatigue most often go away in about two to nine days, but the psychological symptoms may last longer.

The best, most sensible method is to gradually decrease your caffeine and coffee consumption. During this attempt, remember the following:

- Drink six to eight glasses of filtered mineral water each day, which you should buy only in glass bottles, as plastic bottles are petroleum-derived products that contain toxic phthalates.
- Start your day by drinking one to two glasses of noncarbonated mineral water plus one glass of mineral water with freshly-squeezed lemon juice at room temperature.
- Let yourself take a break or a nap when you feel tired.
- Daily, light exercise enables you to warm and loosen up your muscles and overcome fatigue.
- You can find regular relaxation in a warm bath with sea salt. Allow yourself a minimum of twenty minutes for this luxury; a sauna also does the trick.
- Using any sort of relaxation technique is highly recommended, whether it's listening to nature sounds or your favorite music or spending time on your favorite hobby. Every five minutes you spend on relaxation brings wonderful results—after all, the pause button is not just for our electronic gadgets.

I won't say it's easy! I'm quite aware of how hard it is, but I also know that these efforts are worth it, that your body and mind will breathe a sigh of relief and will soon show their gratitude. You'll receive the gift of inner calm; clear thoughts; peaceful, sound sleep; patience; and a healthy perspective on reality. Your emotions will be genuine and balanced, and you'll no longer get irritated or upset for no reason. Your complete health will return and, with it, the desire to live life to its joyful fullest. Its bright sides will finally emerge from the shadows, and healthy, vital energy will enable you to enjoy them.

But what if this experiment fails, and yet another set of promised changes never arrives? Not to worry—I've also got a few tips for that. My aim is not to guilt-trip anyone. Quite the opposite, I want to help even those who have never even considered the possibility of giving up coffee.

- First, don't buy ground coffee. We should always use beans that are freshly ground, ideally right before drinking.
- Coffee should be organic, fair trade, and certified for quality. Coffee is not cultivated in the United States or in Europe; that's why we don't have complete, effective control over the way it's grown. We don't know what or how many protective chemicals, pesticides, or herbicides are used in the regions it comes from.
- The truth is coffee farming is not mechanized, which increases the costs of obtaining the coffee berries and leaves growers unable to afford any losses. The plants are sprayed with chemical agents to achieve the highest

yields possible. This is especially true in places where the berries are harvested only once a year, so that they can remain competitive with regions where the coffee berries ripen twice annually. The contents of nearly every cup of coffee are unknown, and solving this riddle is certainly not in producers' interest.

- Coffee should be consumed as quickly as possible, no more than ten minutes after brewing, since it oxidizes very quickly. Soon, no nutrients remain besides water, caffeine, and … pesticides and herbicides.

- The best, healthiest option is to drink an espresso after a meal.

- Never drink coffee with sugar or milk, since this puts an incredible strain on the body and inflicts untold damage.

- If you have sensitive or overworked adrenal glands, do not drink black coffee. Some sort of fat should be added; this could be butter; fresh, unpasteurized whipping cream; coconut oil or coconut milk; or almond milk. Recall the wise natives of some African regions who chewed their coffee in the form of balls made from the berries' pulp and fat. It was this form that turned out to be the most useful for them.

- Women planning to become pregnant or already expecting should not drink coffee. The research indicates that coffee causes changes to the circulatory system in mothers and the fetus. These include variations in pulse and blood pressure. Caffeine can make it more difficult for women to maintain proper levels of iron and calcium, which is especially critical during pregnancy.

Juice

The list of beverages to avoid is a long one. The most important are pasteurized milk and industrially carbonated and sweetened drinks enriched with a myriad of chemical substances. We should also add fruit juices to the list; they are simply highly concentrated sugar water, since the fruits' vitamins oxidize quickly and are damaged during processing.

A single glass of orange juice has just as much sugar as a candy bar. This sugar is fructose, which is more harmful than refined sugar when deprived of its accompanying vitamins and fiber. Drinking apple juice is tied to developmental disruption in toddlers.[248] Excessive fruit juice consumption upsets the acid balance in the stomach. The presence of the appropriate acids and enzymes in this environment is not only essential for normal digestion but also needed to fight harmful bacteria that could threaten our health.

Although vegetable juices are not as sweet as fruit-based ones, drinking them too often can still have negative consequences. This isn't the only time that exercising moderation and caution can work in our health's favor. The Greek philosopher Euripides would be pleased with such an observation, as he stated, "The best and safest thing is to keep a balance in your life, and to acknowledge the great powers

---

[248] M. M. Smith and F. Lifshitz, "Excess Fruit Juice Consumption as a Contributing Factor in Nonorganic Failure to Thrive," *Pediatrics* 93:3 (1994): 438-443.

around us and in us. If you can do that, and live that way, you are really a wise person."

We know how important healthy, fresh fruits and vegetables are in our daily diet. They are not only incredibly valuable sources of vitamins, macro- and microelements, organic acids, fiber, and many other nutrients, but they offer a variety of flavors, hues, and aromas to our senses, enriching our perception of the world. Nobody would disagree that delicious food brings great pleasure.

But if you find yourself reaching for a vegetable or fruit beverage, remember a few facts.

Around one kilogram (2.2 pounds) of carrots is needed to obtain 170 grams (nearly six ounces, which is less than a full glass) of carrot juice. If these vegetables are the products of conventional farming, you're likely drinking toxic sugar water mixed with a whole host of chemicals, forming a dangerous concoction of pesticides, herbicides, and artificial fertilizers. You must admit that such a drink is a complete contradiction of its imagined health benefits.

Through the strikingly logical, perfect process of evolution, the human body developed mechanisms allowing it to perform all the functions it needs to survive and thrive. In the hypothalamus of the human brain, we can locate the body's "appetite center," which controls our feelings of hunger and satiety. It is easy to see how it works when we eat too many apples, cherries, or grapes. Such an excess of fructose is extremely ill-advised, as can be seen in the instant reactions of our digestive and excretory systems.

These sudden processes irritate the GI tract and cause mineral deficiencies in the body. Fresh, organic, unprocessed fruit consumed in appropriate amounts is not only healthy and beneficial but also delicious. I heartily recommend this method of obtaining nutrients. If, however, you crave fruit or vegetable juices, try to make sure that the raw materials needed to prepare them are of the highest quality, since only that can guarantee their full range of nutrients and flavor.

Juices you have made should be prepared just before drinking to protect their vitamins against oxidation and damage. They should always be diluted with water to reduce their fructose content.

Under no circumstances should you consume industrially produced juices, much less give them to children. This rule should be followed with absolute consistency! Despite glossy advertisements making these juices out to be some sort of nectar, the mythical drink of the gods that brought immortality, they are in fact dangerous liquids whose contents cannot be considered healthy.

Water

I'd like to draw your attention now to the most precious liquid in the universe: water. It seems water is everywhere; many people react with disbelief when they hear there are regions with such a severe lack of water that every drop is worth not its weight in gold but in human lives.

When we learn that the earth's atmosphere holds millions of tons of water vapor,[249] while 20 percent of the planet's fresh water can be found in a single, two-kilometer-deep Siberian lake (Lake Baikal), we might think environmentalists' calls

---

[249] *Wielki ilustrowany atlas świata* [Large Illustrated Atlas of the World], 214.

to save water and warnings that humanity may run out are grossly exaggerated.

Meanwhile, nearly all belief systems consider water to be the "first matter" (*prima materia*), the foundation of all things. A Greek philosopher living at the turn of the sixth century BCE claimed that "everything comes from water, from water it was created and of water it consists" and certainly didn't link this natural phenomenon with the deities Oceanos and Thetis. He observed that "what is alive lives on moisture, and what is dead dries up; the seeds of all things are moist and all nourishment contains juice."[250] So, what role does water play in our bodies? How much do we need to function properly? What kind of water should we drink, and what kind should we avoid?

There are two fundamental factors in human life: water and oxygen. Every chemical process that takes place in our bodies needs water to run. Contemporary medicine is becoming more and more interested in the human body's outstanding capacity for self-healing and water's role in its mechanisms. The body knows how to keep itself in good condition and maintain its youthful vigor. It instinctively senses that, without water, any efforts made are futile and can threaten its existence.

I gave a few pieces of information on this subject at the beginning of this chapter. Now, I'll expand on them with a few more data points. Nearly two-thirds of the human body's mass is water, while the human embryo is around 90 percent

---

[250] Opaliński Władysław, *Słownik symboli*, 475.

water.[251] Our energy levels depend significantly on how much water we drink.

It has been shown that a mere 5 percent decrease in body fluids causes a 25 to 30 percent drop in energy in the average person, while a loss of 20 percent could lead to death! Water is essential for metabolizing fats into useful energy, and it participates in many enzymatic and chemical reactions in the body.

It transports nutrients, hormones, antibodies, and oxygen via our bloodstream and lymphatic system. Proteins and enzymes function more efficiently in less viscous solutions. It is estimated that over 80 percent of the population suffers from energy losses due to slight dehydration. Water helps regulate body temperature via sweat, which cools our bodies and disperses harmful excess heat. It is also necessary to keep our lungs sufficiently moist while we breathe, to prevent them from drying out. We lose anywhere from one to two liters (one to two quarts) of water each day in the process.

The kidneys' filtering function also requires water, since uric acid, urea, and lactic acid must be dissolved in it. When this component is lacking, these substances are not effectively eliminated, which can lead to kidney damage. The kidneys need around 1.5 liters of water a day. When much less is supplied, water is drawn from the intestines, leading to constipation and difficulty passing hard stools.

When we provide our bodies with enough water, we see it best in the appearance and quality of our urine. The urine flows freely from the urinary tract, is a light straw color, and

---

[251] Chlebińska, *Anatomia i fizjologia człowieka* [Human Anatomy and Physiology], 287.

is practically odorless. When the body senses a lack of water, it decreases the amount of urine expelled, while its color and odor become much more intense as the kidneys take up additional fluids to do their jobs. Water is also necessary for proper joint mobility. It works as a moistener and lubricant and is essential for even the slightest activity of the skeletal system.

Obviously, those aren't all the functions of this life-giving liquid, but to name more would go far beyond the scope of this publication. What we should take away from this discussion is never to let our bodies become dehydrated. If you're aware that adults lose nearly two to three quarts of water each day, then the sum of the following data won't come as a shock: we lose anywhere from 100 to 250 grams (3.5 to nearly 9 ounces) of water through the soles of our feet each day, 1 to 2 quarts through breathing, around 1 quart through our sweat (with light physical activity and at a moderate temperature), and from 1 to 1.6 quarts through our urine.

These losses may be higher when playing sports and during intense work, fevers, heat waves, and many other circumstances. Replenishing our body water should be a consistent, daily habit.

Signs of dehydration include feelings of exhaustion, weakness, headache, joint and stomach pain, stomach ulcers, constipation, dry skin, disorientation, slow reflexes, poor concentration, and so on. "Dry" lips are the last external sign of an extreme water deficiency—this means the body may have lost as much as 2 percent of its water content. We should never allow ourselves to stumble into such a situation! Interestingly, thirst is signaled through hunger. Drinking a glass of water is enough to get rid of it. A lack of fluids weakens every aspect of all the biochemical processes taking place in the body.

Water is water! Nothing can take its place—not coffee, not tea, not juice or any other drink. These can't be counted toward our daily water needs! Coffee is a diuretic and dehydrates the body. After drinking one cup of coffee, we should drink three cups of water to make up for the losses it causes.

How do we know how much water we should be drinking every day? There's a very simple formula: just multiply your weight in kilograms by 0.033 to get the number of quarts you need.[252] If I weigh 59 kilograms (130 pounds), that means I should drink 59 x 0.033 = 1.947 quarts of water every day. If you play sports or do some other strenuous physical activity, you should drink more.

When providing water for yourself and the rest of your household, pay attention to some important information. The best water for our health has a hardness level of 170 milligrams per liter or greater and a TDS (total dissolved solids) level of 300 milligrams per liter or greater.[253]

The pH should be between 7 and 8.5. I recommend adding a pinch of sea salt to each glass of water to replenish your electrolytes and further enrich it with beneficial minerals. I'll remind you again that you should only buy water in glass bottles. There are plastic bottles with the special labels #2 HDPE (high-density polyethylene), #4 LDPE (low-density

---

[252] F. Batmanghelidj, *Your Body's Many Cries for Water* (Falls Church, VA: Global Health Solution, 1992).

[253] M. Fox, *Healthy Water* (Portsmouth, NH: Healthy Water Research, 1990, 1998), online at www.healthywater.com.

polyethylene), and #5 PP (polypropylene) that don't release toxic substances, but who wants to remember these awful symbols? Better to go with tried-and-true safe glass bottling!

We shouldn't drink water or any other beverages while eating, since they dilute our stomach acid and put excessive strain on the digestive system. Stomach acid performs all its functions at a pH of one to three. Water can negatively alter this acidity and thereby disrupt the digestion of food in the stomach. We should drink water forty-five minutes to an hour before a meal and forty-five minutes to an hour and a half afterward.

We should also avoid drinks that are too hot or too cold. Neither of these extremes benefits our health. Cold fluids make digestion practically impossible, while high temperatures block enzymes from entering the food we consume. A wonderful morning gift to our bodies, which have become dehydrated during the night, is to drink a half quart of water with a pinch of good sea salt.

Drinks made from milk, fruit, herbs, seeds, and vegetables that have undergone lacto-fermentation are quite healthy and tasty. Lacto-fermentation is a process in which special bacteria transform sugar and starch into beneficial acids. Such beverages are especially good for intestinal problems and blockages, and they also improve digestion, boost energy, help strengthen convalescents, and increase the human body's immunity. They contain many valuable minerals in ionized form along with minimal natural sugars. All of this has wide-reaching benefits for our health and beauty. They are also excellent thirst-quenchers and a treat for the palate to boot.

Wine and Beer

Now, I'd like to share a handful of information on two popular, traditional drinks—wine and beer—and their impact on the body. This information is for those who enjoy and appreciate these drinks, yet find themselves living in a world of myths about them.

As Benjamin Franklin aptly put it, "Wine is constant proof that God loves us and wants to see us happy." The attitude of many world religions toward drinking alcohol has evolved over the centuries, but today generally all of them support either complete abstinence or drinking only in moderation. Ancient evidence of winemaking can be found in many regions of our world, but the most famous comes from the Caucasus—Armenia and Georgia—as well as Iran and Turkey, with scientists dating it back to ca. 8500 BCE.

Today, wine from the most famous vineyards of Bordeaux, Burgundy, Rioja, Languedoc, Alsace, the Rhine Valley, and the Loire Valley can be found on nearly all the tables of the world and compete with Californian, African, and Australian wines.

The controversies over alcoholic drinks will likely never be resolved and will go on for as long as humanity continues to imbibe. In every country and on every continent, these drinks are a source of pleasure but also many problems and misfortunes. However, if we want to drink, it is best to choose biodynamic wine or unpasteurized beer—from small local producers, of course. The predictable appeal to drink responsibly would not be out of place here.

Researchers point out that consuming wine, primarily red wine, can help fight heart disease. There is a well-known, widespread opinion that those who drink moderate amounts of red wine—one to two glasses a day—live longer than both those who overindulge and those who completely abstain.

But is there really something to rejoice in here? The truth is red wine does contain very strong antioxidants, which have been credited with significantly slowing the aging process and which are also found in the skin of fresh grapes. These substances activate a type of protein—sirtuin—which is considered to have rejuvenating capabilities. A single glass of wine, however, is not enough to initiate this process, and the amount necessary to do so would undoubtedly damage our livers. With an unhealthy liver and damaged brain, regaining our youth is highly unlikely. Alcohol always has a negative effect on our brain cells, irreversibly destroying them.

The ancients drank wine diluted with water at a ratio of 1:1 or 1:4. The actual alcohol content of such a beverage was quite low. Many traditional societies known for their longevity continued this practice for centuries. They consumed moderate amounts of alcohol, mainly light wine and beer made from grapes, bananas, or other fruit. The Roman writer and government worker Pliny the Elder (living in the first century CE) dedicated the entire fourteenth chapter of his encyclopedic *Natural History* to the topic of wine, discussing its benefits and warning against consuming it in excess.

If you decide wine isn't your thing and you don't have any reason to drink it (after all, its health benefits are doubtful and its overpromoted flavonoids can be found in many fruits and vegetables), you can absolutely eliminate it from your diet without any pangs of conscience or have just a glass or two during a nice dinner with friends or family. Personally, I don't deny myself this pleasure, since I also believe that "wine is constant proof that God loves us and wants to see us happy," and I want God to see me happy! Let it be God's will, and let's drink to that!

As the old Polish saying goes, "Wine in the belly is strength in the spirit." So, we can have a glass or two when the daily grind robs us of our strength and the peace and quiet we so desire. Euripides noted in *The Bacchae*, "Where there is no wine, there is no love." We shouldn't merely take him at his word—but allow ourselves a little experimentation.

Now, let's take a closer look at a drink that is just as popular as wine: beer. Many global consumers don't even count it as alcohol! I won't comment on whether that's due to ignorance or hypocrisy. In many cultures, beer is considered a manly drink, since it is men who make up the clear majority of its consumers.

Unfortunately, beer enthusiasts are easy to spot, even without any specialist equipment and without being a medical expert. Male lovers of this beverage often sport large, distended bellies that spill over their pants, over which hang their ample, almost-female breasts.

This occurs because beer contains large amounts of hops, making it the most estrogen-rich drink we know. This plant is the most powerful plant source of estrogen, the female hormone. German beer producers and hops growers noticed long ago how young women harvesting hops matured more quickly and began menstruating earlier than peers who did not work on such crops.

A mere 100 grams of hops contain anywhere from thirty to three hundred thousand IUs of estrogen, depending on the variety.[254] This is primarily in the form of estrogen known as estradiol, which, once it enters the male body, causes a radical drop in the level of testosterone—the male hormone. It also interferes with Leydig cells, which are responsible for the production of this hormone in the testes. The conclusion to be drawn from this discussion is clear—male beer lovers can reduce their libido significantly!

My aim is not to urge you to give up these beverages but to pay attention to how much you drink and to keep it under conscious control. It's worth it to stand up to popular opinion, live healthily, and persevere in your search for your own divine nectar.

Remember

- We should completely give up sweetened and carbonated beverages.
- Fruit and vegetable juices from large producers labelled "100% natural" are in fact 100 percent artificial products having nothing in common with healthy drinks.
- Two cups of black, unsweetened coffee a day is an acceptable amount.

---

[254] "Beer, Hops, Estrogen, Sedation of the Population—Why Men Shouldn't Ever Drink Beer," *Lifetwink*, last updated March 10, 2012, http://lifetwink.com/ beer-hops-estrogen-sedation-of-the-population-men-shouldnt-ever-drink-beer/.

- Fresh fruits and vegetables are healthier than the juices made from them, since they contain beneficial fiber and do not contain as much condensed fructose.
- A healthy adult should drink high-quality water, in an amount calculated using the following formula: 0.033 x your body weight (in kilograms).
- Coffee, tea, cocoa, or other drinks do not count toward our daily water needs—these beverages do not ensure the right level of water in our bodies.
- Neither water nor other drinks should be consumed during meals, as they dilute the stomach acid and put an excessive strain on the digestive system.
- Beer is alcohol, and it not only intoxicates its male drinkers but also delivers an uncontrolled dose of estrogen that diminishes their sexual prowess.
- Many myths surround wine that are not born out in reality; wine is more a social lubricant than a health-promoting beverage.

CHAPTER 18

A REVIEW OF TEMPTING DIETS

Statisticians say each of us devours around one ton of food each year. What's in that ton? Are we nourishing ourselves properly? Are there optimal ways of using up all the nutrients in our food? What should we eat to be beautiful, healthy, and youthful and to live long and happy lives? Such questions can go on forever, and we could search for the answers for ages without the hope of ever finding even one that would fully satisfy our curiosity.

There seem to be many sources of information. Just pick up any glossy magazine, browse the store window displays, or listen to interviews with yet another celebrity, star, or idol to see for yourself how hot this topic is, how far-reaching, and how … uncertain. The publications that tackle these issues are endless. The next time you go to a bookstore or browse around on the Internet, make sure to spend some time learning more about this field. Every few months, I find myself lingering by the health and lifestyle section at the bookstore to see what's new and what they're trying to sell today as part of the latest and "best," "most effective," "revolutionary" new diet, which represents a complete break with all diets known and promoted before.

The publishing market currently offers thousands of diet books, with new ones popping up all the time. If the advice they contained had any bearing on reality, we should now be the strongest, healthiest, most beautiful and sculpted generation in the history of humankind.[255]

Unfortunately, I think we all can see how far the authors' assurances are from the truth. The value of the global health market is estimated at hundreds of billions of dollars, a large part of which is from this literature, which serves as an effective promotional tool for specific food products, dietary supplements, or drinks. The system also harnesses the power of the media, celebrities, scientists, and especially the research institutions that analyze these diets.

Let's take a closer look at this process, since specific figures are always the best illustration of people's interest in the problem of obesity and our means of fighting it. Weight loss and weight management are big business. The global market is expected to reach $206.4 billion by 2019, growing from $148.1 billion in 2014 at a compound annual growth rate of 6.9 percent from 2014 to 2019.[256]

As a more specific example, Americans spend over $60 billion on weight loss every year! This figure is the result of systematic growth in national spending on this goal. In 2008,

---

[255] People, particularly millennials, seem more focused on health—especially for purposes of vanity—than ever before, which will change the trajectory of this issue in the present.

[256] "Global Weight Loss and Weight Management Market 2015–2019—Fitness Equipment, Surgical, Diet and Weight Loss Services Analysis," PR Newswire, last updated April 23, 2015, http://www.prnewswire.com/news-releases/global-weight-loss-and-weight-management-market-2015-2019-fitness-equipment-surgical-diet-weight-loss-services-analysis-300071062.html.

that figure was $58.6 billion; in 2009, it was $60.4 billion; and in 2010, it was $60.9 billion.[257] The statistics also state that around 50 percent of Americans and British people are trying to lose or maintain their weight, and 108 million adult Americans were on a diet in 2012![258] Unfortunately, all the effort and money they spent on achieving or maintaining a proper weight turned out to be in vain, as the research also shows that nearly everyone who goes on a diet (90 to 95 percent) eventually returns to his or her previous weight or gains weight over the following one to five years.

Kevin Hall, a scientist at a US federal research center, followed contestants from the reality TV show *The Biggest Loser* for six years after their final weigh-ins in 2009. The study was the first to measure what happened to people over a longer period after losing significant amounts of weight through intensive dieting and exercise. The stunning results showed just how hard the body resists heavy weight loss.[259] Most of the season's contestants regained most if not all the weight they lost; some are even heavier now.[260] Unfortunately, almost everything we think of as commonsense solutions to obesity and weight loss—just eat less and exercise more!—are myths regularly challenged by science.

[257] "Diet and Weight Loss Statistics," FitnessforWeightLoss.com, accessed June 18, 2015, http://www.fitnessforweightloss.com/diet-and-weight-loss-statistics.

[258] Marketdata Enterprises Inc., "Number of American Dieters Soars to 108 Million; Market to Grow 4.5% to $65 Billion in 2012" (Press Release).

[259] Nancy LeTourneu, "What the $60 Billion Weight Loss Industry Doesn't Want You to Know," *Washington Monthly*, accessed May 20, 2017, http://washingtonmonthly.com/2016/05/02/what-the-60-billion-weight-loss-industry-doesnt-want-you-to-know/.

[260] Gina Kolata, "After *The Biggest Loser*, Their Bodies Fought to Regain Weight," *New York Times*, accessed May 20, 2017, https://www.nytimes.com/2016/05/02/health/biggest-loser-weight-loss.html.

Of course, this phenomenon doesn't just apply to Americans on reality TV shows; the problem of obesity is now becoming increasingly global. In view of the unsettling rise in the number of people struggling with obesity—35 percent of adults and 17 percent of children and adolescents—on June 19, 2013, the AMA (American Medical Association) in Santa Monica, California, officially announced a new health policy meant to fight this phenomenon. Obesity was officially recognized as a disease requiring treatment and a series of medical interventions.[261]

There are an astonishing number of diets, and they all spark heated debates on their quality and effectiveness. All of them, however, take advantage of readers' ignorance and desperation, often showing only the brighter side of the ideas that accompanied their creation and popularization. Also, most of the big diet plans sell their own food, which is loaded with chemicals and preservatives and not at all nutritious.

The time has come to take control of your health and life and exercise this control responsibly on your own. Buddha's advice may prove useful in this endeavor: "Renounce evil deeds, cultivate good ones, and control your mind." We should rediscover the old, lost path that kept the body in good condition.

Food should not be a dire problem, in which all the joy in our meals comes hand in hand with a fear of obesity or anxiety over introducing the toxins it holds into our bodies.

---

[261] Jacque Wilson, CNN, "Physicians Group Labels Obesity a Disease," updated June 19, 2013, http://edition.cnn.com/2013/06/19/health/ama-obesity-disease-change/index.html.

We shouldn't let food become an obsession. Eating should be a pleasure and a joy, not a punishment.

The human body knows and can signal precisely what it needs; after all, it has survived for millennia without dieticians' advice. The human body survived famine, extreme weather conditions, threats posed by predators, and constant attacks by viruses, bacteria, and parasites, as well as many other adverse factors. Our ancestors developed effective systems of control, balance, immunity, and energy replenishment that would not only guarantee their survival but also their strength and fitness, so as to produce offspring and ensure their safety. We should make use of their priceless experience.

Remember

- Our emotional states and the types of our emotions have a remarkable impact on how well our organs function.
- Negative feelings, such as sadness, pessimism, worry, and distrust, disrupt our digestion and impair the functioning of the spleen, stomach, liver, and pancreas.
- Anger, jealousy, vindictiveness, and hatred increase "bad" cholesterol levels and hinder our bodies' ability to remove toxins and produce bile.
- Fear disrupts the normal workings of the kidneys and bladder. It lowers your sex drive and causes desperation and a loss of interest in life.
- Even the best-planned diet cannot bring results in our bodies if we allow ourselves to go through life full of negative emotions.

CHAPTER 19

WHERE TO BEGIN

Long ago, Heraclitus pondered the origins of nature and its properties. The Greek philosopher, living at the turn of the fifth century BCE, found its fundamental attribute to be change. He took a river to be a symbol of this change, hence the well-known sayings "Everything flows; nothing stands still" and "You can't step in the same river twice." These nuggets of wisdom became a metaphorical picture of reality in constant flux, in which stagnation is merely an illusion. In this eternal motion—the flow of all things—nothing is permanent, nothing absolute.

We should actively and consciously join in this transformative process and help build the reality surrounding us as well as ourselves. Most of us have such a need for active change; we just have to discover it and know how to use it to our advantage. Every new beginning is difficult, and sometimes the mere thought of change—with the image of the enormous effort that allegedly comes along with it—can stress us out, terrify us, or discourage us from taking that first step. But if you consider change to be as natural to life as breathing, if you consider its presence as a sign of progress and of being one step closer to becoming your best self, nothing will stand in your way. Just try to do only those things that you can achieve honestly and without stress now, without introducing any radical changes or chaos into your life. If your first step is simply drinking enough water and adding a few more fresh vegetables, that's absolutely fine. If you add a short daily walk or two into your routine a bit later, no worries—that's exactly where you should start.

You'll see that the more out-of-balance your body was, the unhealthier your lifestyle at the outset, the more careful, slow, and subtle you'll need to be to dig yourself out of this situation. Don't treat yourself to any kind of shock therapy! Such radical measures won't bring you relief, improvement, or release from your previous problems.

Making sudden large, revolutionary changes to many different aspects of your life at once becomes another source of additional, unnecessary stress—an excellent way to hamper or even thwart your plans to become healthy. The pace at which you should introduce changes to guarantee comfortable, surefire results and a peaceful transition period is different for everyone. But it should never cause excessive discomfort or involve heavy sacrifices. Of course, you should count on a bit of unpleasantness, which may worry or even discourage you at the beginning. There's no such thing as a free lunch! But this small price shouldn't end up being an irreparable loss, ruining your previous subjective world, draining your accounts, and negating all your life's work up to now. This path of change is a road leading to harmony, openness to positive effort, knowing your own limits, and the conscious taking of your fate into your own hands—a road you should set out to travel with joy.

Where there's a will, there's a way. So as you look for motivation, repeat to yourself and your children and loved ones the beautiful, inspiring words of the renowned Spanish cellist, Pablo Casals:

> Each second we live is a new and unique moment of the universe, a moment that will never be again ... Do you know what you are? You are a marvel. You are unique ... You may become a Shakespeare, a Michelangelo, a Beethoven ... You must work, we must all work, to make the world worthy of its children.[262]

Remember

- Each person has an inexhaustible wealth of ability, talent, and skill that he or she can draw upon to grow as a person and achieve his or her goals.
- The body and mind work in synergy as two parts of the same system and exert an enormous influence on all aspects of human functioning. Treating them as separate entities will never give us a full, thorough, and realistic picture of humankind.
- Knowing your own self-worth is fundamental to feeling well, satisfied, and true to yourself as you play all your roles in your family, professional life, school, and society.

---

[262] "MusicUnitesUs, Public School Education Program," Brandeis University, accessed May 28, 2017, http://www.brandeis.edu/musicunitesus/education/.

DIETARY DESIDERATA (FIFTEEN COMMANDMENTS)

1. Our lives are based on the energy and life found in our food. Fresh food contains many active enzymes. These enzymes are like a spark, without which you couldn't light even the feeblest flame. Highly processed, lifeless food forces the body into a state of stagnation. The food we eat should be fresh, organic, and locally grown. Try to make sure it is unprocessed or minimally processed before it's eaten.

2. Eat when you're hungry, and stop when you're full. Finish your meal when you feel satisfied, not when you're full to bursting. Overeating is just as harmful as undereating. Your brain doesn't receive the satiety signal and eliminate your feeling of hunger until twenty minutes after you've finished your meal.

3. Relax during meals. Food should be eaten in a pleasant, calm atmosphere. By turning off the TV and avoiding heated discussions, you'll avoid digestive issues and appreciate the taste, fragrance, and wonderful appearance of the dishes served.

4. Eat local, seasonal products. The changes in season guarantee a marvelous variety of foods to consume. We should take advantage of this natural offering. Seasonal food appears when it is of the highest quality, at the peak of freshness and at its greatest nutritive value.

5. Don't be a pack rat—go shopping often! Shop for fresh products at least twice a week; don't let them accumulate in the fridge or pantry. Purchase amounts that you can eat relatively quickly, without leaving your food to wilt, go bad, or get freezer burned.

6. Become a snob—only buy products that are organic and ecofriendly. Traditionally farmed plants contain much higher levels of antioxidants, minerals, and vitamins than those cultivated as part of large commercial crops awash in chemical agents. Organic production protects the soil and water and treats animals humanely. These aren't the slogans of some "green" ecofanatics or commercial swindlers but an absolute rule of life for those wise enough to take responsibility for themselves! If such people are snobs—*then be a snob!*

7. Eat as many vegetables as you can and limited amounts of fruit. Fresh, organic fruits and vegetables are true treasure troves of minerals and vitamins. They boast valuable fiber and phytochemical substances that protect us from cancer, heart disease, and many other devastating illnesses. The fiber from fruits and

vegetables is essential to the proper functioning of many processes in the digestive system. If too much of our fiber comes solely from cereal grains, this leads to nutritional deficiencies, since cereals block the absorption of nutrients and interfere with the digestive system's elimination of waste.

8. Eat only high-quality animal protein from organically raised creatures and small, wild saltwater fish, which are marked by their high levels of EPA and DHA omega-3 fatty acids.

9. Be suspicious of white foods; in fact, it's best to avoid them altogether. White flour, white sugar, white salt, and milk that has been pasteurized and homogenized should be taken off our shopping list. If you want certain products and you can't find raw, ecofriendly ones, opt for those labelled as certified organic.

10. If you can't figure out what's in a product without a chemical dictionary and magnifying glass—don't eat it! It's not good for your eyes, your knowledge, or (especially) your liver.

11. Season your food with sea salt (e.g., Celtic sea salt), Himalayan salt (which looks like tiny amethyst crystals), or New Zealand salt, since they contain many valuable microelements and almost no heavy metals.

12. Never forget that without water, life is impossible. Drink 1.5 to 2 liters of this priceless, life-giving liquid

each day. Don't try to cheat and count tea, juice, beer, or coffee as water. *Water is water*, and nothing can replace it. If you don't have access to a natural, tested water source, then buy the best brands on the market. Check to see that the bottles haven't been overheated or left to stand in the sun or by the heater. In such cases, the water can become contaminated with toxins from plastic bottles. The easiest solution is to drink water from glass containers, adding a pinch of sea salt to enrich it with additional minerals.

13. Give up harmful foods that make you feel bad after eating them, since this has a destructive impact on your health.

14. Following a proper diet for your metabolic type and changing your habits and lifestyle are more pleasant and easier than continually taking medications now or in the future. When we keep such important aspects of our daily functioning in mind, we can avoid or reduce this risk to the very minimum. Try to eliminate the causes of an illness, not its symptoms.

15. Live according to the 80:20 principle, which should be interpreted in the following optimistic way: if you take care of yourself sensibly and responsibly 80 percent of the time, the remaining 20 percent can be spent indulging yourself and joyfully exclaiming, "You only live once! Let the good times roll!"

APPENDIX A

Mini Cheat Sheets

Get Your Fats Right

Healthy fats are those that are rich in nutrients and have fed numerous generations over thousands of years. All of them should come from small, noncommercial, certified organic farms. Sometimes your friends' small farms may not have such certificates. This does not preclude you from buying the food they produce, so long as their sanitary conditions and means of growing crops and raising animals seem trustworthy, and careful observation of and conversations with the farmers gives us enough reliable information.

Good Fats for Cooking that Are Susceptible to High Temperatures (Saturated Fats)

- They are most often found in a solid state.
- They harden at low temperatures.
- They deliver a concentrated form of energy to the body.
- They do not easily go rancid when heated to high temperatures.
- They are found in butter and clarified butter.

- They include beef and lamb tallow, pork lard, and poultry fats (chicken, goose, and duck).
- They are found in coconut and palm oil.

Good Fats for Cold Salad Dressings (Monounsaturated Fats)

- These fats are liquid at room temperature.
- They do not go rancid too quickly.
- They should be extra virgin or first cold-pressed and always come in a dark glass container. After opening, they should be used quickly or stored in the refrigerator for a short time; it is best to buy them in small amounts, so we know they are fresh. They include olive oil (can also be used for cooking, but only for up to four minutes and at low temperatures), sesame and nut oils, flaxseed/linseed oil, and avocado oil.

Good Fats Enabling Proper Dissolution of Fat-Soluble Vitamins (Polyunsaturated Fats)

- These fats contain omega-3 linolenic acid and omega-6 linoleic acid, both of which are essential for our bodies, which cannot produce them.
- They remain in liquid form even when frozen.
- They should never be heated.
- They spoil very easily.
- They include fish liver oils, e.g., cod liver oil (better than fish oils, which do not provide fat-soluble vitamins, can lead to excessive levels of unsaturated fatty acids, and usually come from farm-raised—and thus toxic—fish).

Eat Plenty of Good Fats!

- Use organic butter made from raw, grass-fed milk instead of margarines and vegetable oil spreads.
- Use coconut, ghee, or lard for cooking. They are much better than any other cooking oils and are loaded with health benefits.
- It is better to use olive oil cold, drizzled over salad or fish, for example. It is not an ideal cooking oil, as it is easily damaged by heat.
- Be sure to add healthy fats to your diet, such as avocados; raw dairy products; raw nuts, such as almonds, pecans, and macadamia nuts; seeds; unheated organic nut oils; grass-fed meats; organic egg yolks; and olive oil. Also take a high-quality source of animal-based omega-3.

Fats to Be Absolutely Avoided!

- These include hydrogenated and partially hydrogenated oils (trans fats, trans isomers, and hardened vegetable oils). They are produced in a process known as partial hydrogenation from the cheap oils of such plants as corn, sunflowers, cotton seeds, soybeans, canola, and safflower seeds. Because of the ease of use, transport, and storage of solid fats in the food industry (and technology), a special method of so-called hardening and refining liquid fats is used to change plant oils (and fish oil) into solid fats through hydrogenation, after which fragrances, water with NaCl, powdered milk, emulsifiers, colorings, and vitamins (most often A and

E) are added. Such fat is (unfortunately!) widely used in the food processing industry.

All of the following fats (which are, in fact, toxic plastics) can cause cancer, heart disease, immune system dysfunction, infertility, difficulty concentrating, osteoporosis, growth problems, clogged arteries, and so on:

- industrially processed liquid soybean, canola, safflower, corn, and cottonseed oils
- margarine and vegetable butter
- vegetable fats and oils that can be heated to very high temperatures when baking and frying
- fats from industrially raised animals—these are highly toxic and exceptionally harmful because of the use of hormones, antibiotics, and pharmaceuticals to treat or vaccinate the herd; these chemical substances accumulate in the fat of these animals and later make their way into our bodies along with our food
- fats with a prolonged shelf life (ability to store for a long period)—they contain numerous substances to slow the rancidity process, synthetic vitamins and minerals to replace the natural ones lost in processing, and chemical substances to improve the fats' taste, color, and appearance
- artificial *trans* fats (created in an industrial process that adds hydrogen to liquid vegetable oils to make them more solid), which can be found in French fries, fried chicken, doughnuts, cakes, cookies, crackers, bread, chips, pretzels, breaded and fried foods, and

ready-made salad dressings and mayonnaise—most bars and restaurants fry their food and prepare their sauces using only these fats

Get Your Sugar Right

It's easy to make a mistake in the world of sugars and sweeteners, yet the lives of consumers lost in this world are certainly not sweet. To help you find your way, I've put together a summary of all the sugars available on the market. But the essential tip remains the same, and I'll continue to repeat it like a mantra: read the labels!

- Dextrose, fructose, and glucose are simple sugars. The fundamental difference between them is the way they are metabolized by our body. Some sugars are easily dealt with by our body, while others cause many difficulties. Glucose and dextrose are essentially the same, yet producers use the term *dextrose* more often when describing a food item on its label.
- Corn syrup, which contains 55% fructose and 45% glucose, should never be consumed.
- Sugar alcohols (xylitol, glycerol, sorbitol, maltitol, mannitol, and erythritol) are neither sugars nor alcohols but are becoming more widely used as sweeteners. They cause digestive problems, including bloating, diarrhea, and gas. They should not be consumed.
- Sucralose is advertised with the misleading slogan "Made from sugar," but, in fact, it is an artificial, chlorinated sweetener just like aspartame and saccharin.

It's extremely harmful! You should never consume it! In fact, sucralose was discovered by accident while developing a new insecticide and was never intended for human consumption.

- Honey is 53 percent fructose, but it is completely natural in its unprocessed, raw form. Raw honey offers many undeniable health benefits. Three teaspoons of honey a day will keep ten doctors away! When used in moderation, it is indispensable to our body. I am a big supporter of honey. I wholeheartedly recommend it to everyone, although those three teaspoons are a bit excessive; I suggest one a day as a healthy and sufficient amount. My personal favorite is New Zealand manuka honey, which creates an inhospitable environment for bad bacteria in the gut.

- Agave nectar is 95 percent fructose! It is falsely advertised as a natural product. Actually, agave nectar is so highly processed that the final product in no way resembles the original, natural agave plant. We can avoid adding it to our diet without any qualms!

- Stevia is a very sweet plant native to South America. The sweetener made from its leaves is completely safe and tasty. I recommend it as a nutritious alternative. Not all stevia products are created equal. The best option is green leaf stevia, and while stevia extracts are acceptable, avoid altered stevia blends. By the time a product like this is placed on a shelf, very little of the stevia plant remains.

- Luo han (luohanguo) is a natural sweetener produced from monk fruit, which, along with coconut sugar, I can also recommend with a clean conscience. Both are healthy, sweet, and contain tons of vitamins. I'd also like to draw your attention to coconut sugar, which makes a delicious addition to desserts, ice cream, gelatin, and so on.

A List of Substances Hazardous to Your Health (and Life)

If a food item has even one of the following poisons in its ingredients, it absolutely should not find its way onto your table:

- preservatives: sodium benzoate, sodium nitrite, potassium sorbate, BHA, BHT, TBHQ
- sweeteners and sugar substitutes: fructose, corn syrup, aspartame (E951), sucralose, acesulfame K (E950)
- food colorings: FD&C Blue No. 1 and 2, FD&C Green No. 3, FD&C Red No. 3 and 40, FD&C Yellow No. 5 and 6, Orange B, Citrus Red No. 2
- artificial flavors: ethyl formate (rum fragrance), ethyl acetate (pear fragrance), ethyl butyrate (banana fragrance)—these are primarily used to produce aromatic essences that are widely used in the production of confectionery products, dairy products (flavored yogurts and kefirs), juices, dessert drinks, and fruit-flavored gelatin
- flavor enhancers: monosodium glutamate (MSG; E621), hydrolyzed soy protein, yeast extract, glycine

and its sodium salt (E640), maltol (E636), ethyl maltol (E637), and calcium inosinate (E633)

A description of a few of these may help you understand how toxic the substances we unwittingly encounter are.

- BHA and BHT: carcinogenic organic compounds that secretly poison our organs—found in breakfast cereals, mixed nuts, chewing gums, butter, meat, potato chips, and beer
- rBHG and rBST: synthetic hormones responsible for breast, colon, and prostate cancer; most often found in milk and dairy products
- arsenic: classified as a human carcinogen by the EPA; found in poultry
- food coloring agents: Blue 1 and 2, Yellow 5 and 6—most food colorings are obtained from coal tar, which is carcinogenic; they are used mainly in the confectionery industry to produce cakes, cookies, candy, and cake decorations and are also used to color pasta, cheeses, medications, sport and energy drinks, and animal food
- azodicarbonamide—causes asthma and disrupts the breathing process; found in bread, frozen dinners, pasta mixes, and packaged baked goods (cookies, corn puffs, pretzels, and so on)

I realize this mini cheat sheet looks more like a secret list of deadly poisons being used to kill off humankind. Rest assured, however, that this is an incomplete selection representing just a small percentage of the toxins present in the food available in markets around the world. Obviously, then, money spent on healthy, chemical-free, and organic food is not wasted. After all, not all products are created equal!

A fresh, fragrant apple from the orchard that has not been sprayed with any toxic substances is a vitamin bomb. But once these organic factors are taken away, it can become a chemical bomb, insidiously depriving us of our health. Another unacceptable threat is posed by consuming products of uncertain origin. This concerns all types of food: grains, fruit, vegetables, fats, and meats. Everything depends on the *quality* of a given product, where it comes from, and the conditions under which it was created.

Our knowledge on this subject can change the corrupt global economic structures of unhealthy food producers. How? The answer is simple: we stop buying their products! Let this be more than just a declaration! Each of us should systematically and consistently put it into practice.

Boycott items that have

- an extremely long shelf life
- numerous ingredients
- labels with unclear information
- labels with information written in such fine print that you need a magnifying glass to read it
- labels with chemical names, symbols, and numerical designations

APPENDIX B

Perfect Oatmeal Recipe[263]

This is an old-fashioned one, but it is easy to follow. There is no slaving over a hot stove for hours. A little preparation is all you need. Try it; you'll love it.

Ingredients

1 cup of rolled organic oats
1 cup of water
a pinch of sea salt
1 teaspoon of unpasteurized cider vinegar
1 cup butternut squash puree (optional)
1 heaping tablespoon of organic butter (be generous here)
1 teaspoon of raw honey
1/2 an apple, grated
1/2 a handful of chia seeds
a few walnuts
1 teaspoon of cinnamon

---

[263] Barbara Rubin, "Perfect Oatmeal Recipe," https://www.barbararubin.org/archives/3948.

Preparation

Soak the oats in just enough water to cover them. Add the sea salt and cider vinegar. Leave overnight. The next morning, drain the oat/salt/vinegar mixture and rinse thoroughly. Add fresh water, again enough to cover the oats, and bring the oat/water mixture to a boil. Use medium-plus heat. Add butternut squash puree. Turn the heat down to low-medium, and stir until the oatmeal is as thick as you want it. You can add water if you like your oatmeal more on the runny side. Remove the cereal from the heat, and add the butter and honey. Cover and let the mixture rest for about 5 to 10 minutes. Add the apples, seeds, and walnuts (you can substitute different fruit, seeds, and nuts if you like), cinnamon and any other ingredients that will make your oatmeal extra tasty. You can add yogurt or kefir, or you can have a lovely meal by adding more honey. Get creative!

Perfect Chicken Broth Recipe[264]

The following recipe is healthy, inexpensive, and easy to follow. A few chops with a knife and that's all there is to it. One small housekeeping item before you begin, though. Get the best organically raised, pasture- or grass-fed chicken (or rooster) you can find. Animals that are raised in confined spaces, fed synthetic diets, or given drugs will not provide you with optimal benefits. Do not scrimp here. Get an

---

[264] Barbara Rubin, "Baby It's Cold Outside!" https://www.barbararubin.org/archives/851.

additive-free animal, and use organic vegetables. Your broth will taste better for it!

Ingredients

4 quarts (or more) water (You want the chicken to be completely covered.)
2 tablespoons raw apple cider vinegar
1 large onion, coarsely chopped (organic)
2 carrots, peeled and coarsely chopped (organic)
3 celery stalks, coarsely chopped (organic)
1 whole free-range chicken (or 2 to 3 pounds of chicken parts, bone-in). If you can get your hands on a rooster, that would be even better.
2–4 chicken feet (This is optional, but a great addition. The feet of the chicken are rich in sulfur, a mineral that is critical for brain function and that helps in the extraction of gelatin from the bones of the chicken.)
3–5 laurel leaves
10 allspice leaves
1 large handful of parsley (organic)

Preparation

Fill a large pot with filtered water. You will be cooking this for a long time, so you may want to use a crockpot. Add the raw vinegar, onions, carrots, and celery. Add the chicken. Bring the mixture to a boil (uncovered), and remove any scum that rises to the top. Reduce the heat to its lowest setting. Once the mixture is simmering, add in the laurel leaves and allspice and cover the pot. If you have used a whole chicken or chicken parts that have meat on them, the meat will begin to separate from the bones after about 2 hours. Remove the meat, and continue to let the mixture simmer for at least 7 hours. You can let it heat for up to 24 hours. Just make sure it does not burn. Remove the bones with a slotted spoon. Then, add in the fresh parsley, and let the mixture continue to simmer for about 10 minutes. This will add extra nutrients and flavor to your broth. Finally, let the broth cool in the refrigerator overnight. A layer of fat will rise to the surface. Skim this off. You can save it for frying.

Tip—whenever I make a batch of chicken broth, I actually double the recipe and freeze some for later use.

Have fun and stay healthy!
—Barbara

GLOSSARY

acidic. Having the properties of an acid, or containing acid; having a pH below 7.

adrenal fatigue. A term applied to a collection of nonspecific symptoms, such as body aches, fatigue, nervousness, sleep disturbances, and digestive problems. The term often shows up in popular health books and on alternative medicine websites, but it isn't an accepted medical diagnosis.

adrenal glands. Located at the top of each kidney, the adrenal glands produce hormones that help the body control blood sugar, burn protein and fat, react to stressors like a major illness or injury, and regulate blood pressure. Two of the most important adrenal hormones are cortisol and aldosterone.

alkaline. Something that is alkaline contains an alkali or has a pH value of more than 7.

alpha-tocopherol. Vitamin E.

aluminosilicate minerals. A group of minerals that contain the compounds alumina (Al_2O_3) and silica (SiO_2), hence the name aluminosilicate. Alumina and silica are two of the most common compounds in the earth's crust, and, as a result, they form some of the most common minerals on earth. Many gemstones, including emeralds, are aluminosilicates.

amine. A compound in which one or more of the hydrogen atoms in ammonia have been replaced by an organic functional group.

amylase (ptyalin). An enzyme in the saliva that converts starch into sugar.

amylopectin A. A type of carbohydrate found in starch that we commonly consume, such as from rice, potatoes, and bread.

angiotensin. A protein hormone that causes blood vessels to become narrower.

anthropological. Relating to the study of humankind.

anthropology. The science that deals with the origins, physical and cultural development, biological characteristics, and social customs and beliefs of humankind.

antioxidants. Substances that may protect cells in your body from free radical damage that can occur from exposure to certain chemicals, smoking, pollution, and radiation and as a by-product of normal metabolism.

archaeology. The scientific study of material remains (such as tools, pottery, jewelry, stone walls, and monuments) of past human life and activities.

arginine. An essential amino acid and a key component of protein. Lack of arginine in the diet impairs growth, and in adult males, it decreases the sperm count. Arginine is available in turkey, chicken, and other meats and as L-arginine in supplements.

ascorbic acid. A vitamin found particularly in citrus fruits and green vegetables. It is essential in maintaining healthy connective tissue and is also thought to act as an antioxidant.

aspartame. An artificial sweetener used as a sugar substitute in some foods and beverages.

aspartic acid. A nonessential amino acid, meaning the body can manufacture enough of this amino acid in the liver from food sources. However, aspartic acid does play a major role in metabolism.

astaxanthin. A naturally occurring carotenoid found in algae, shrimp, lobster, crab, and salmon. Carotenoids are pigment colors that occur in nature and support good health.

atherosclerosis. A disease in which plaque builds up inside your arteries. Arteries are blood vessels that carry oxygen-rich blood to your heart and other parts of your body. Plaque is made up of fat, cholesterol, calcium, and other substances found in the blood.

autism. A mental condition, present from early childhood, characterized by great difficulty in communicating and forming relationships with other people and in using language and abstract concepts.

avitaminosis. A condition resulting from a deficiency of a particular vitamin.

beriberi. A disease causing inflammation of the nerves and heart failure, ascribed to a deficiency of vitamin B1.

beta-carotene. A red-orange pigment found in many fresh fruits and vegetables.

bifidogenic effect. Promoting the growth of (beneficial) bifidobacteria in the intestinal tract.

bioavailable. A drug or other substance entering the circulation when introduced into the body and so able to have an active effect.

biocatalyst. A substance, especially an enzyme, that initiates or modifies the rate of a chemical reaction in a living body.

biochemical processes. Processes that occur in living organisms. For example, the way your body converts food into energy is biochemical, as is the way your body fights disease and responds to drugs.

biodiversity. The variety of plant and animal life in the world or in a particular habitat, a high level of which is usually considered to be important and desirable.

biodynamic. Agriculture is a form of alternative agriculture very similar to organic farming, but it includes various esoteric concepts drawn from the ideas of Rudolf Steiner.

bioflavonoids. Any of a group of water-soluble yellow compounds present in citrus fruits, rose hips, and other plants. Bioflavonoids are antioxidants.

caffeol. A volatile oil in coffee beans, giving the characteristic flavor and aroma.

carbohydrates. Mainly sugars and starches, together constituting one of the three principal types of nutrients used as energy sources (calories) by the body. Carbohydrates can also be defined chemically as neutral compounds of carbon, hydrogen, and oxygen.

carbon dioxide. A colorless, odorless gas produced by burning carbon and organic compounds and by respiration. It is naturally present in air (about 0.03 percent) and is absorbed by plants in photosynthesis.

carcinogens. A substance capable of causing cancer in living tissue.

carotene. An orange or red plant pigment found in carrots and many other plant structures.

carotenoid. Any of a class of mainly yellow, orange, or red fat-soluble pigments, including carotene, which give color to plant parts, such as with ripe tomatoes and autumn leaves.

casein. A milk protein present in the milk from all mammals. It is found in dairy products, such as cheese, milk, and yogurt.

catalysis. Specialized chemistry to make a chemical reaction happen or happen more quickly.

cell membranes. Also known as the plasma membrane, a double layer of lipids (fat) and proteins that surrounds a cell and separates the cytoplasm (the contents of the cell) from its surrounding environment.

cell receptor. A protein molecule that receives chemical signals from outside a cell.

cerebral cortex. The largest region of the cerebrum in the mammalian brain, it plays a key role in memory, attention, perception, cognition, awareness, thought, language, and consciousness.

chelation. A type of bonding of ions and molecules to metal ions.

chlorination processes. The process of adding chlorine (Cl_2) or hypochlorite to water. This method is used to kill certain bacteria and other microbes in tap water, as chlorine is highly toxic.

cholesterol. A substance containing a lot of fat that is found in the body tissue and blood of all animals.

choline. A water-soluble nutrient that is related to other vitamins, such as folate and vitamin B. Just like B vitamins, choline plays a similar role in terms of supporting energy and brain function, as well as keeping the metabolism active.

chorea. Rapid, violent movements of the muscles that are difficult to stop or control.

citric acid monohydrate. A key intermediate in metabolism. It is an acid compound found in citrus fruits.

cochineal red (E124). A food additive approved by the European Union (EU). It is used as a synthetic coloring agent in food and drink products.

coenzymes. A substance that enhances the action of an enzyme.

collagen. The main structural protein found in skin and other connective tissues.

colostrum. A yellowish liquid, especially rich in immune factors, secreted by the mammary gland of female mammals a few days before and after the birth of their young.

conjugated linoleic acid (CLA). An unsaturated fatty acid in the milk and meat of cows, sheep, and goats.

cortisol. A steroid hormone that is produced by the adrenal glands, which sit on top of each kidney. When released into the bloodstream, cortisol can act on many different parts of the body and can help your body respond to stress or danger, increase your body's metabolism of glucose, and control your blood pressure.

cranium. The hard bone case that gives an animal's or a human's head its shape and protects the brain.

cystic fibrosis. A hereditary disease that causes the body to produce thick and sticky mucus that can clog the lungs and obstruct the pancreas.

DDT. One of the first chemicals in widespread use as a pesticide.

dextrose. A natural form of sugar that is found in fruits, honey, and in the blood of animals.

DHA (docosahexaenoic acid). An omega-3 fatty acid that is a primary structural component of the human brain, cerebral cortex, skin, and retina.

DHEA. A steroid hormone made by the adrenal glands that acts on the body much like testosterone and is converted into testosterone and estrogen.

disaccharides. Also called a double sugar, a disaccharide is a molecule formed by two monosaccharides or simple sugars. Three common disaccharides are sucrose, maltose, and lactose.

embolism. A blocked artery caused by a foreign body, such as a blood clot or an air bubble.

encephalization. Defined as the amount of brain mass related to an animal's total body mass. An animal's encephalization has been argued to be directly proportional, although not equal, to that animal's level of intelligence.

endocrine system. The collection of glands that produce hormones that regulate metabolism, growth and development, tissue function, sexual function, reproduction, sleep, and mood, among other things.

endorphin. A chemical naturally released in the brain to reduce pain that, in large amounts, can make you feel relaxed or full of energy.

enzyme. A protein that functions as a catalyst to mediate and speed a chemical reaction.

EPA (eicosapentaenoic acid). A fatty acid found in the flesh of cold-water fish, including mackerel, herring, tuna, halibut, salmon.

epicure. A person who enjoys high-quality food and drink.

epigenetics. The study of biological mechanisms that will switch genes on and off.

ergocalciferol. Vitamine D2.

erythrocytes (hemolysis). Red blood cells that travel in the blood.

estradiol. A form of the hormone estrogen.

estrogen. A hormone that is important for sexual and reproductive development, mainly in women. It is also referred to as the female sex hormone.

ethanol (ethyl alcohol). Grain alcohol and drinking alcohol.

evolutionary biology. The study of the changes in the characteristics of a species over several generations through the process of natural selection.

extracellular fluid. Denotes all body fluid outside the cells.

flavonoids. A diverse group of phytonutrients (plant chemicals) found in almost all fruits and vegetables. Along with carotenoids, they are responsible for the vivid colors in fruits and vegetables.

folic acid. A vitamin of the B complex found especially in leafy green vegetables, liver, and kidney.

free glutamic acid (MSG). One of the most abundant amino acids. It can occur naturally in some foods, but more often, it is an artificial chemical construct riddled with contaminants used as a flavor enhancer.

free radicals. Atoms that contain one or more unpaired electrons. Free radicals are believed to be a cause of aging, heart disease, and some cancers.

gene. The part of a cell in a living thing that controls its physical characteristics, growth, and development.

ghrelin. The "hunger hormone," it plays a key role because it signals your brain to eat. Ghrelin is a hormone produced in the gut.

GI tract. The gastrointestinal tract consists of a hollow muscular tube starting from the oral cavity, where food enters the mouth, continuing through the pharynx, esophagus, stomach, and intestines to the rectum and anus, where food is expelled.

gliadins. A glycoprotein (a carbohydrate plus a protein) within gluten.

gluconeogenesis. A metabolic pathway that results in glucose formation in animals from a noncarbohydrate source, as from proteins or fats. It takes place mostly in the liver, though it can also happen in smaller amounts in the kidney and small intestine.

glucose. A simple sugar that is an important energy source in living organisms and is a component of many carbohydrates.

glutamine. An important amino acid, L-glutamine is the form found in foods, supplements, and the human body. It is part of the proteins in your body and involved in immune function and intestinal health.

glutathione. Often referred to as the body's master antioxidant. Composed of three amino acids—cysteine, glycine, and glutamate—glutathione can be found in virtually every cell of the human body. The highest concentration of glutathione is in the liver, making it critical in the body's detoxification process.

glycemic response. The effect that food has on blood sugar (glucose) levels after consumption.

glycine. An amino acid, a building block for protein. It is not considered an "essential amino acid" because the body can make it from other chemicals.

glycogen. The stored form of glucose that the body warehouses for future use. It is stored mainly in the liver and the skeletal muscles.

glycoproteins. Simply proteins with a sugar attached to them.

goitrogen. A medical term that is used to describe any substance that interferes with function of the thyroid gland. (The **thyroid gland** is a butterfly-shaped organ located in the base of your neck. It releases hormones that control metabolism—the way your body uses energy.)

hemoglobin. The protein molecule in red blood cells that carries oxygen from the lungs to the body's tissues and returns carbon dioxide from the tissues back to the lungs.

5-HIAA. A urine test that measures the amount of *5-hydroxyindoleacetic acid*. 5-HIAA is a breakdown product of a hormone called serotonin. This test tells how much serotonin is in the body.

homocysteine. An amino acid that is produced by the human body.

homocysteine levels. An abnormal accumulation of **homocysteine**, which can be measured in the blood, can be a marker for the development of heart disease.

hormones. A chemical substance produced in the body that controls and regulates the activity of certain cells or organs.

Huntington's disease. Also known as Huntington's chorea, Huntington's disease is an inherited disorder that results in the death of brain cells.

hydrogenate liquid oils. Hydrogenation is the chemical process by which liquid vegetable oil is turned into solid fat.

hyperacidity. A condition in which the level of acid in the gastric juices is excessive, causing discomfort.

hypervitaminosis. A condition of abnormally high storage levels of vitamins, which can lead to toxic symptoms.

hypoglycemia. Also known as low blood sugar, hypoglycemia is when blood sugar decreases to below normal levels. This may result in a variety of symptoms, including clumsiness, trouble talking, confusion, loss of consciousness, seizures, or death.

hypothalamus. A part of the brain that has a vital role in controlling many bodily functions, including the release of hormones from the pituitary gland.

hypovitaminosis. A condition produced by lack of an essential vitamin.

ileum. The last and narrowest part of the small intestine.

indoctrination. The process of teaching a person or group to accept a set of beliefs uncritically.

intrinsic factor. A substance secreted by the stomach that enables the body to absorb vitamin B_{12}. It is a glycoprotein.

isocaloric. Having similar caloric values.

isomers. Two molecules with the same molecular formula that differ structurally. Therefore, isomers contain the same number of atoms for each element, but the atomic arrangement differs.

isometabolic. This means we can eat one hundred calories of glucose (from a potato or bread or other starch) or one hundred calories of sugar (half glucose and half fructose), and they will be metabolized differently and have a different effect on the body.

lactase. An enzyme that breaks down the milk sugar lactose into glucose and galactose.

lactic acid. An acid that exists in sour milk and is produced in muscles after a lot of exercise.

Lactobacillus. A rod-shaped bacterium that produces lactic acid from the fermentation of carbohydrates.

lactose. The sugar found in milk.

lecithin. A substance found in plant and animal tissue, often used in food products to help the different parts mix together well.

leptin (the starvation hormone) a peptide hormone that is produced by fat cells that plays a role in body weight regulation by acting on the hypothalamus to suppress appetite.

Leydig cells. Produce the hormone testosterone, which is vital for sperm production. They are found inside male testicles, next to the seminiferous tubules, where sperm are produced.

melatonin. A hormone that is produced by the pineal gland and is intimately involved in regulating the sleeping and waking cycles, among other processes.

membrane. A microscopic double layer of lipids (fat) and proteins forming the boundary of cells or organelles.

Mendeleev's periodic table. A table in which the chemical elements are arranged in order of increasing atomic number. Elements with similar properties are arranged in the same column (called a group), and elements with the same number of electron shells are arranged in the same row (called a period).

metabolic effect. Relating to metabolism, the whole range of biochemical processes that occur within us (or any living organism).

metabolism. The chemical processes that occur within a living organism in order to maintain life.

methane. The main constituent of natural gas.

methanol. A light, volatile, flammable poisonous liquid alcohol. CH_3OH is used especially as a solvent, antifreeze, or denaturant for ethanol and in the synthesis of other chemicals.

methylmercury. An organic form of mercury that is highly toxic and is the main culprit in mercury poisoning.

monosaccharides (glucose, fructose). The simplest units of carbohydrates and the simplest form of sugar.

morphine. A powerful narcotic agent that has strong analgesic (pain relief) action and other significant effects on the central nervous system. It is dangerously addictive.

mucous membranes. The thin skin that covers the inside surface of parts of the body, such as the nose and mouth, and produces mucus to protect them.

mycotoxin. A toxic substance produced by a fungus and especially a mold.

NAFLD, or non-alcoholic fatty liver disease. A very common disorder referring to a group of conditions where there is an accumulation of excess fat in the liver of people who drink little or no alcohol.

niacin. One of the B complex vitamins found in foods such as wheat, beef, chicken, and milk, important for producing energy from food and for keeping the digestive and nervous systems healthy.

nitrates. Inorganic compounds made up of nitrogen and oxygen, NO_3 (one nitrogen and three oxygen molecules). These compounds combine with other elements like sodium and potassium to make sodium nitrate or potassium nitrate. They are used as preservatives and color fixatives in cured meats and have other industrial uses, such as in gunpowder, explosives, fertilizers, and glass enamels.

nitric oxide (NO). A colorless, poisonous gas, NO is formed by the oxidation of nitrogen or ammonia that is present in the atmosphere; paradoxically, it plays a number of important roles in the body.

nitrogen. A colorless, odorless, unreactive gas that forms about 78 percent of the earth's atmosphere.

nitrosamines (N-nitroso). Present in various food products, they are carcinogenic in laboratory animals.

oligosaccharides. Any carbohydrate of from three to six units of simple sugars (monosaccharides).

paleontology. A science dealing with the life of past geological periods as known from fossil remains.

pancreatic enzymes. Enzymes that help break down fats, proteins, and carbohydrates.

pancreatic islets. Also called islets of *Langerhans*, tiny clusters of cells scattered throughout the pancreas.

pancreatitis. Inflammation of the pancreas.

papain. A protein-digesting enzyme obtained from unripe papaya fruit, used to tenderize meat and as a food supplement to aid digestion.

parotid glands. The parotid gland is one of the three salivary glands contained within the human body. The same applies to many animals. It is the largest of the three glands, as well as the biggest producer of saliva.

pathogens. A bacterium, virus, or other microorganism that can cause disease.

pellagra. A disease caused by a deficiency of niacin in the diet, characterized by skin changes, severe nerve dysfunction, mental symptoms, and diarrhea.

pepsinogen. A substance that is secreted by the stomach wall and converted into the enzyme pepsin by gastric acid.

peptones. A soluble protein formed in the early stage of protein breakdown during digestion.

pesticide. A substance used for destroying insects or other organisms harmful to cultivated plants or to animals.

phagocytes. A type of cell in the body that can surround things and swallow them, especially a white blood cell that protects the body against infection by destroying bacteria.

phthalates or phthalate esters. Esters of phthalic acid. They are mainly used as plasticizers, i.e., substances added to plastics to increase their flexibility, transparency, durability, and longevity.

phytoestrogen. A substance found in certain plants that can produce effects like that of the hormone estrogen when ingested into the body.

phytonutrient. A substance found in certain plants that is believed to be beneficial to human health and help prevent various diseases.

phytosterols (referred to as plant sterol and stanol esters). A group of naturally occurring compounds found in plant cell membranes. Because phytosterols are structurally similar to the body's cholesterol, when they are consumed, they compete with cholesterol for absorption in the digestive system.

pituitary gland. The main endocrine gland, it is a small structure in the head. It is called the master gland because it produces hormones that control other glands and many body functions, including growth.

platelet adhesion. The clumping together of platelets in the blood. Platelet aggregation is part of the sequence of events leading to the formation of a thrombus (clot).

polyphenols. One of the most important and certainly the most numerous among the groups of phytochemicals present in the plant kingdom.

polysaccharide. A large molecule made of many smaller monosaccharides (starch, cellulose). Monosaccharides are simple sugars, like glucose.

proline. An amino acid that is a constituent of most proteins, especially collagen.

protein. One of the many substances found in food such as meat, cheese, fish, or eggs that is necessary for the body to grow and be strong.

provitamin. A substance that is converted into a vitamin within an organism.

reactive oxygen species (ROS). A type of unstable molecule that contains oxygen and that easily reacts with other molecules in a cell. A buildup of reactive oxygen species in cells may cause damage to DNA, RNA, and proteins and may cause cell death. Reactive oxygen species are free radicals. Also called an oxygen radical.

renin. An enzyme secreted by the kidneys that plays an important part in the maintenance of blood pressure by activating angiotensin, a hormone that causes the constriction of blood vessels, which increases blood pressure.

retinal hemorrhage. A disorder of the eye in which bleeding occurs into the light-sensitive tissue on the back wall of the eye.

retinol. An animal form of vitamin A.

riboflavin. A yellow vitamin of the B complex that is essential for metabolic energy production.

rickets. A deficiency disease that affects the young during the period of skeletal growth. It is characterized especially by soft and deformed bones and is caused by failure to assimilate and use calcium and phosphorus normally because of inadequate sunlight or vitamin D.

scurvy. A disease caused by a lack of vitamin C and characterized by spongy gums, loosening of the teeth, and bleeding into the skin and mucous membranes.

serotonin. A chemical that has a wide variety of functions in the human body. It is sometimes called the happy chemical, because it contributes to well-being and happiness.

shelf life. The length of time that a product, especially food, can be kept in a shop before it becomes too old to be sold or used.

single-gene disorder. When a certain gene is known to cause a disease, we refer to it as a single-gene disorder or a Mendelian disorder.

sirtuin. A protein that regulates cell metabolism and aging.

squalene. An oily liquid hydrocarbon that occurs in shark liver oil and human sebum and is a metabolic precursor of sterols. Squalene is used in skincare products as a highly effective emollient and natural antioxidant. Historically, they've been used in the medical field to treat wounds and skin problems.

stachyose (raffinose and verbascose). Nondigestible carbohydrates mainly found in beans.

stearic acid. A substance like wax that is used for making candles and for some medicines and saturated fats.

sybarite. A person who loves expensive things and pleasure.

T cell. A type of white blood cell. T lymphocytes are part of the immune system and develop from stem cells in the bone marrow.

testosterone. The key male sex hormone that regulates fertility, muscle mass, fat distribution, and red blood cell production.

theobromine. A bitter component closely related to caffeine that occurs especially in cacao beans and has stimulant and diuretic properties.

thyroid. A gland that makes and stores hormones that help regulate the heart rate, blood pressure, body temperature, and the rate at which food is converted into energy.

tocopherol. Any of a group of fat-soluble alcohols that occur in wheat-germ oil, watercress, lettuce, egg yolk, and so on. They are thought to be necessary for healthy human reproduction. Also called vitamin E.

triglycerides. A type of fat found in the blood. High levels of triglycerides may raise the risk of coronary artery disease.

uric acid. A product produced by the body after the purines in many foods undergo the digestive process and are broken down inside the body. After this breakdown process, the uric acid travels through the bloodstream into your kidneys, and most is actually eliminated through the urinary tract via urination.

vasculitis. Inflammation of a blood vessel or blood vessels.

vasoconstriction. Narrowing of the blood vessels that results from contraction of the muscular walls of the vessels. The opposite of vasoconstriction is *vasodilation*.

zonulin. A protein that modulates the permeability of tight junctions between cells of the wall of the digestive tract.

BIBLIOGRAPHY

Aleksandrowicz, Julian, and Irena Gumowska. *Kuchnia i medycyna [Cooking and Medicine]*. Warsaw: Watra, 1991.

Awdiejew, Aleksy. "O wegetarianizmie" [On Vegetarianism]. *Charaktery 5 no. 52 (May 2001): 49.*

Axe, Josh. *Eat Dirt: Why Leaky Gut May Be the Root Cause of Your Health Problems and 5 Surprising Steps to Cure It.* New York: HarperCollins Publishing, 2016.

Bennett, Peter, Stephen Barrie, and Sara Faye. *Dieta oczyszczająca [Seven-Day Detox Miracle]*. Warsaw: Diogenes, 2003.

Bochenek, Krystyna, and Darek Kortko. "Rzuć palenie! Rozmowa z prof. Witoldem Zatońskim z Centrum Onkologii w Warszawie" [Quit smoking! A Conversation with Prof. Witold Zatoński of the Maria Skłodowska Curie Memorial Cancer Centre in Warsaw]. Gazeta Wyborcza, November 17, 2009, Duży Format. http://wyborcza.pl/duzyformat/1,127290,1775966.html.

Brillat-Savarin, Anthelme. *Fizjologia smaku [The Physiology of Taste]*. Warsaw: PJW, 1977.

Brückner, Aleksander. *Encyklopedia staropolska [Encyclopedia of Old Poland]*, vol. I. Warsaw: Księgarnia Trzaski,

Everta i Michalskiego, 1937. Reprint, Warsaw: PWN, 1990, 572.

Calton, Jayson, and Mira Calton. Rich Food Poor Food. Malibu, CA: Primal Blueprint Publishing, 2013.

Challem, J. J. "Beta-Carotene and Other Carotenoids: Promises, Failures and a New Vision." Journal of Orthomolecular Medicine 12, no. 1 (1997): 11–19.

Chek, Paul. How to Eat, Move and Be Healthy. San Diego: C.H.E.K. Institute, 2004.

———. The Last Four Doctors You'll Ever Need—How to Get Healthy Now! C.H.E.K. Institute. Multimedia ebook.

Chlebińska, Janina. Anatomia i fizjologia człowieka [Human Anatomy and Physiology]. Warsaw: Wydawnictwa Szkolne i Pedagogiczne, 1975.

Chwalba, Andrzej. Obyczaje w Polsce [Customs in Poland]. Warsaw: Wydawnictwo PWN, 2004.

Clement, Brian. Supplements Exposed. USA: New Page Books, 2010.

Cordain, Loren. The Paleo Diet. Hoboken, New Jersey: John Wiley & Sons, Inc., 2002.

Cruise, Jorge. Metoda 100: licz tylko cukrowe kalorie i schudnij 9 kg w 2 tygodnie [The 100 Method: Count Only Sugar Calories and Lose Up to Eighteen Pounds in Two Weeks]. Warsaw: Grupa Wydawnicza Foksal, 2013.

Datner, Szymon, and Kamieńska, Anna. Z mądrości Talmudu [From the Wisdom of the Talmud]. Warsaw: PIW, 1988.

Davis, William. Wheat Belly Total Health. New York: Rodale, 2014.

De Leth, Richard. OERsterk. The Netherlands: Uitgeverij De Leth, 2012.

Doroszewski, Witold. *Słownik języka polskiego* [*Dictionary of the Polish Language*]. Warsaw: PAN, 1958.

Enig, Mary, and Sally Fallon. *Eat Fat Lose Fat*. New York: Penguin Group, 2006.

Faigin, Rob. *Natural Hormonal Enhancement*. Cedar Mountain, NC: Extique Publishing, 2000.

Fallon, Sally, and Mary Enig. *Nourishing Traditions*. Washington: New Trends Publishing, 2007.

Fitzgerald, Randall. *The Hundred-Year Lie: How Food and Medicine Are Destroying Your Health*. New York: Penguin Group, 2006 (ebook).

Fromm, Erich. *The Sane Society*. London and New York: Routledge Classics, 2002.

———. *Zdrowe społeczeństwo* [*The Sane Society*]. Kraków: Vis-à-Vis/Etiuda, 2012.

Fukuyama, Francis. *Koniec człowieka. Konsekwencje rewolucji biotechnicznej* [*Our Posthuman Future: Consequences of the Biotechnology Revolution*]. Kraków: Wydawnictwo Znak, 2004.

Gittleman, Ann-Louise. *Beyond Pritikin*. New York: Bantam Books, 1980.

Głosik, Jerzy. *Przygoda z archeologią* [*Adventures in Archeology*]. Warsaw: Nasza Księgarnia, 1987, 69–119.

Grodecka, Maria. *Wszystko o wegetarianizmie* [*All about Vegetarianism*]. Katowice and Warsaw: Vega Katowice/SPAR Warszawa, 1991.

Heizer Wharton, Charles. *Ten Thousand Years from Eden*. Orlando: WinMarkPublishing, 2001.

Hellerman, Caleb. "No Scientific Evidence Diet Supplements Work." *CNN*, 2007. http://edition.cnn.com/2007/HEALTH/04/06/chasing.supplements/.

Hildegard of Bingen. *Sensacje i porady na każdy dzień [Sensations and Advice for Every Day]*. Poznań: KSW, 1998.

Historia sztuki świata [History of World Art]. Joint publication. Warsaw: Muza SA, 1998. 14–21.

Howell, Edward. *Enzyme Nutrition*. USA: Avery Publishing Group, 1985.

Hutt, Joachim, and Helmut Klein. *Potrawy biblijne [Dishes of the Bible]*. Kraków: WAM, 2005.

Johnson, Richard J., and Timothy Gower. *The Sugar Fix: The High-Fructose Fallout That Is Making You Fat and Sick*. New York: Pocket Books, 2009.

Kalish, Daniel. *Your Guide to Healthy Hormones*. USA: Natural Path, 2005.

Kitowicz, Jędrzej. *Opis obyczajów za panowania Augusta III. [A Description of Customs during the Reign of Augustus III]*. Wrocław: Zakład Narodowy im. Ossolińskich, 1970, 453–456.

Kopaliński, Władysław. *Słownik symboli [Dictionary of Symbols]*. Warsaw: Wiedza Powszechna, 1990.

Kumat, Stanisław. *Niech się staną bogowie [Let There Be Gods]*. Warsaw: Nasza Księgarnia, 1963.

Künstler, Mieczysław J. *Sprawa Konfucjusza [The Case of Confucius]*. Warsaw: Iskry, 1983.

Łanowski, Jerzy. *Antologia anegdoty antycznej [Anthology of Ancient Anecdotes]*. Wrocław: Ossolineum, 1970.

Lemnis, Maria, and Henryk Vitry. *W staropolskiej kuchni i przy polskim stole* [Old Polish Traditions in the Kitchen and at the Table]. Warsaw: Wydawnictwo Interpress, 1989.

Levenstein, Harvey. *Paradox of Plenty*. New York: Oxford University Press, 1993.

———. *Revolution at the Table*. New York: Oxford University Press, 1988.

Lipski, Elizabeth. *Digestive Wellness: Strengthen the Immune System and Prevent Disease through Healthy Digestion*. 4th ed. New York: McGraw Hill, 2012.

Lipton, Bruce. *The Biology of Belief*. UK: Hay House, 2008.

Lurker, Manfred. *Słownik obrazów i symboli biblijnych* [Dictionary of Biblical Images and Symbols]. Poznań: Pallottinum, 1989.

Maćko, Anna. "Nie o tym, jak ciężko pracujemy, ale o tym, jak pracujemy ciężko" [It's Not How Hard We Work, but How We Work Hard]. *Charaktery* 56 no. 9 (September 2001), 29–31.

Marseille, Jacques, and Nadeije Laneyrie-Dagen, eds. *Dzieje ludzkości. Największe wydarzenia w historii świata* [The History of Humankind: The Greatest Events in World History]. Presov: Larousse, 2000, 12–22.

Niebrzydowski, Leon. *O poznawaniu i ocenie samego siebie* [On Getting to Know and Assessing Yourself]. Warsaw: Nasza Księgarnia, 1976.

Partyka-Żurowska, Dorota. "W mrocznej jaskinie Lascaux" [In the Dark Cave of Lascaux]. www.euduseek.interklasa.pl/artykuly/artykul/ida/1653/.

Pawlaczyk, Bogusław, and Małgorzata Zakrzewska. *Biblia a medycyna* [*The Bible and Medicine*]. Poznań: KSW, 1998.

Pismo Święte Starego i Nowego Testamentu. Biblia Tysiąclecia [*The Millennium Bible: Holy Scriptures of the Old and New Testament*]. Poznań/Warsaw: Pallottinum, 1971.

Pollan, Michael. *The Omnivore's Dilemma*. Great Britain: Bloomsbury Publishing, 2011.

Prehistoria [Prehistory]. Encyklopedia historyczna świata [*Encyclopedia of World History*], vol. 1. Kraków: Agencja Publicystyczno-Wydawnicza Opres, 1999. 501–511.

Ravnskov, Uffe. *The Cholesterol Myths*. Washington, D.C.: New Trends Publishing, 2000.

———. *Fat and Cholesterol Are Good for You*. Sweden: GB Publishing, 2009.

Rodowicz, Iga. Kuchnia japońska [*Japanese Cuisine*]. Warsaw: Wydawnictwo Tenten, 1991.

Shimek, Ronald. "The Toxicity of Some Freshly Mixed Artificial Sea Water." *Reefkeeping Online Magazine*, 1999. http://www.reefkeeping.com/issues/2003-03/rs/feature/.

Sisson, Mark. *The Primal Blueprint*. Malibu, CA: Primal Nutrition, 2009.

Stukonis, Monika. "Czy ciało to ja?" [*Am I My Body?*]. Twój Styl no. 2/175 (2005): 30–36.

Sudolski, Zbigniew. Krasiński. Opowieść biograficzna [*Krasiński: A Biography*]. Warsaw: Ludowa Spółdzielnia Wydawnicza, 1977, 205–207.

Szuchiewicz, Włodzimierz. Huculszczyzna [*Hutsul Country*]. Warsaw: Grafika/Gopher U.R.P., 2011. Photo-offset reprint of the 1908 edition from the collections of the Warsaw Public Library.

Tatarkiewicz, Władysław. *Historia filozofii* [*History of Philosophy*]. Warsaw: PWN, 1958.

Tokarski, Jan. *Słownik wyrazów obcych* [*Dictionary of Foreign Phrases*]. Warsaw: PAN, 1980.

Traczyk, Władysław. *Fizjologia człowieka z elementami fizjologii stosowanej i klinicznej* [*Human Physiology with Elements of Applied and Clinical Physiology*]. Warsaw: Wydawnictwo Lekarskie PZWL, 2009. 262.

Unterman, Alan. *Encyklopedia tradycji i legend żydowskich* [*Encyclopedia of Jewish Traditions and Legends*]. Warsaw: Książka i Wiedza, 2003.

Urbański, Marek. *Kuchnia chińska* [*Chinese Cuisine*]. Warsaw: Wydawnictwo TEN, 1991.

Walcott, William, and Trish Fahey. *The Metabolic Typing Diet*. New York: Broadway Books, 2000.

Wielki ilustrowany atlas świata [*Large Illustrated Atlas of the World*]. Warsaw: GeoCenter International, 1993, 146–149.

Williams, Roger. *Biochemical Individuality*. USA: Keats Publishing, 1989.

Wilson, James. *Adrenal Fatigue: The 21st Century Stress Syndrome*. Petaluma, CA: Smart Publications, 2001.

Winniczuk, Lidia. *Ludzie, zwyczaje i obyczaje starożytnej Grecji i Rzymu* [*People, Traditions, and Customs of Ancient Greece and Rome*]. Warsaw: PWN, 2006.

Wolfe, David. *The Food and Medicine of the Future*. Berkeley, CA: North Atlantic Books, 2009.

Wrzesiński, Kazimierz. "Cena stresu" [The Price of Stress].
Charaktery (April 2000), 19–20.
Zieliński, Krzysztof. Słownik pochodzenia nazw i określeń
medycznych [Dictionary of the Origins of Medical Names
and Terms]. Bielsko-Biała: A-medica Press, 2004.

Websites

http://chekinstitute.com
http://drhyman.com
http://foodmatters.tv
http://www.drsinatra.com
http://www.drweil.com
http://www.hungryforchange.tv
http://www.mercola.com
http://www.westonaprice.org

Blogs

http://agendafin.com/category/food and drink/coffee/
http://pl.wikipedia.org/wiki/Kawa
http://pl.wikipedia.org/wiki/Ludność_świata
http://pl.wikipedia.org/wiki/Teresa_Neumann
http://pl.wikipedia.org/wiki/Kwas_fitowy
www.korektazdrowia.pl/wp.../prof-witold-zatonski-rola-
prewencji
http://www.lascaux.culture.fr/#/fr/00.xml
http://gadzetomania.pl/7201,oscillococcinum-nie-istnieje
http://cudaswiata.pl/azja/terakotowa_armia.html   (Łukasz
Wieczorek, published August 15, 2008)

http://www.odchudzanko.pl/porady-i-artykuly/nadwaga-i-otylosc/informacje-o-otylosci/statystyki-otylosci-w-polsce-i-na-swiecie/

http://www.ekologia.pl/wiadomosci/srodowisko/polacy-w-pierwszej-dziesiatce-otylych-narodow,16286.html

muzyka.interia.pl/wiadomość dnia/news/dieta-cud-karla-lagerfelda, 224135

http://articles.mercola.com/sites/articles/archive/2000/04/02/vegetarian-myths.aspx

http://articles.mercola.com/sites/articles/archive/2013/07/06/grass-fed-beef.aspx

http://articles.mercola.com/sites/articles/archive/2012/02/02/dutch-recognize-saturated-fat-not-a-problem.aspx

http://articles.mercola.com/sites/articles/archive/2010/08/10/making-sense-of-your-cholesterol-numbers.aspx

http://articles.mercola.com/sites/articles/archive/2013/06/22/food-pyramid-guide.aspx

http://articles.mercola.com/sites/articles/archive/2010/04/20/sugar-dangers.aspx#_edn1

http://articles.mercola.com/sites/articles/archive/2010/04/03/are-you-getting-the-right-type-of-omega3-fats.aspx

http://drrajivdesaimd.com/tag/theories-of-obesity/

http://products.mercola.com/organic-beef/

http://medischcontact.artsennet.nl/actueel/nieuws/nieuwsbericht/113364/veel-artsen-weten-van-wetenschapsfraude.htm

http://www.thincs.org/news.htm

http://www.westonaprice.org/health-topics/the-oiling-of-america/

http://www.theheartfoundation.org/heart-disease-facts/heart-disease-statistics/

http://drrajivdesaimd.com/tag/theories-of-obesity/

http://www.cdc.gov/heartdisease/facts.htm
http://www.cbn.com/cbnnews/healthscience/2012/october/
   cholesterol-myth-what-really-causes-heart-disease/
http://www.ncbi.nlm.nih.gov/pubmed/89498/
http://americannutritionassociation.org/newsletter/hidden-
   hazards-milk (Volume 36 (4))
http://www.livestrong.com/article/264767-how-is-excess-glucose-
   stored/
http://www.pharmacytimes.com/publications/issue/2012/
   October2012/Insulin-Resistance-Recognizing-the-
   Hidden-Danger
http://www.rightdiagnosis.com/i/insulin_resistance/stats-
   country.htm
http://www.hindawi.com/journals/jtr/2011/152850/
http://www.huffingtonpost.com/dr-mark-hyman/wheat-
   gluten_b_1274872.html
http://www.nlm.nih.gov/medlineplus/ency/article/002473.htm
http://www.drpepi.com/aluminum-poisoning.php
http://www.medicinenet.com/mercury_poisoning/article.htm
http://www.westonaprice.org/vitamins-and-minerals/
   the-salt-of-the-earth
http://www.sittingsolution.com/articles/01/?pub=240086&
   hit=321687015&delay=no
http://www.reefkeeping.com/issues/2003-03/rs/feature/
http://www.healthychild.com/synthetic-or-natural-vitamins-
   whats-the-difference/
http://www.nlm.nih.gov/medlineplus/ency/article/002473.htm
http://drhyman.com/about/2012/07/01/10-reasons-to-quit-your-coffee/

http://zdrowie.gazeta.pl/Zdrowie/1,101460,10740117,
Najbardziej_otyle_narody_w_Europie____Polacy
_w_pierwszej.html
http://www.snowvillecreamery.com/a1-and-a2-beta-casein-in-cow-milk.html
http://articles.mercola.com/sites/articles/archive/2013/11/04/saturated-fat-intake.aspx
https://en.wikipedia.org/wiki/Bovine_somatotropin
http://www.jillcarnahan.com/2013/07/14/zonulin-leaky-gut/
https://www.ncbi.nlm.nih.gov/pmc/articles/PMC2607002/
https://oldearthproject.wordpress.com/tag/food-chain/
http://www.abc.net.au/news/2017-07-25/egg-producer-snowdale-holdings-fined-over-free-range-claims/8741706
https://www.aspca.org/shopwithyourheart/advocate-resources/usda-organic-label-and-farm-animal-welfare
https://www.hobbyfarms.com/why-pastured-pigs-are-better/
https://www.aspca.org/animal-cruelty/farm-animal-welfare/animals-factory-farms
https://www.washington.edu/wholeu/2014/06/02/antibiotic-free-meats/
http://humanorigins.si.edu/evidence/human-fossils/species/australopithecus-afarensis

DVDs

Colquhoun, J., and C. Ledesma. Food Matters. Australia: Permacology Productions, 2008.
Colquhoun J., C. Ledesma, and L. Ten Bosch. Hunger for Change. Australia, 2012.

Hunt, C. J. In Search of the Perfect Human Diet. USA: Hunt Thompson Media, LLC, 2012.

Kenner, R. Food, Inc. Hong Kong: Robert Kenner Films, Participant Media, 2009.

Lightning Source UK Ltd.
Milton Keynes UK
UKHW020347190319
339415UK00005B/262/P